HEALTH, HAPPINESS, AND LONGEVITY

Health, Happiness, and Longevity

Eastern and Western Approach

by SUKHRAJ S. DHILLON, Ph. D.

Japan Publications, Inc.

Published by JAPAN PUBLICATIONS, INC.

Distributors:
UNITED STATES: *Kodansha International/USA, Ltd., through Harper & Row, Publishers, Inc., 10 East 53rd Street, New York, N.Y. 10022.* SOUTH AMERICA: *Harper & Row, Publishers, Inc., International Department.* CANADA: *Fitzhenry & Whiteside Ltd., 150 Lesmill Road, Don Mills, Ontario M3B 2T6.* MEXICO AND CENTRAL AMERICA: *HARLA S. A. de C. V., Apartado 30–546, Mexico 4, D. F.* BRITISH ISLES: *International Book Distributors Ltd., 66 Wood Lane End, Hemel Hempstead, Herts HP2 4RG.* EUROPEAN CONTINENT: *Boxerbooks, Inc., Limmatstrasse 111, 8031 Zurich.* AUSTRALIA AND NEW ZEALAND: *Book Wise (Australia) Pty. Ltd., 101 Argus Street, Cheltenham Vic. 3192* THE FAR EAST AND JAPAN: *Japan Publications Trading Co., 1–2–1, Sarugaku-cho, Chiyoda-ku, Tokyo 101.*

First Printing: May 1983

ISBN 0–87040–527–6

Printed in U.S.A.

Preface

A large segment of people are passionately looking for health, happiness, and longevity. These intelligent and well-educated people often end up in a state of confusion to seek help. In health, nutrition, exercise or aging, as in other areas of science, we find many different views. The intelligent approach one would often choose is to follow the views presented by a qualified person, mostly a physician or a scientist. We know that a majority of the physicians are trained for diagnosis of diseases and for prescribing medicine to cure it. We certainly need well-trained physicians to treat sick people, but this disease-related training is quite an opposite of health or vitality or longevity. As far as scientists are concerned, their views are often based on individual experiments, the results of which may display disparities. As discussed further in the Introduction, scientific experiments have many positive effects and I do not want to give a wrong impression about the validity of scientific research. However, a particular set of experiments do not and perhaps cannot, take into consideration all possible complications that may set in, due to the inherently complex nature of biological systems.

The above facts have been clearly realized by most of the health conscious generation of today. The proof for which exists in worldwide popularity of holistic health approaches. Most of the holistic approaches are based on ancient experiences of the eastern world. They are good, natural and less likely to cause side effects. However, many of these need evaluation for their validity in view of western scientific knowledge. The need to incorporate the ancient knowledge of the eastern world and the scientific experimentation of the western world was one of the primary factors that motivated me for writing this book.

Before proceeding further, I must put a word of *caution* here. This is a health book based on preventive approach, and is not presented for the purpose of treating people with serious illnesses. If you have any kind of medical problem and are on drugs, you qualify as a patient requiring a physician's monitoring. There is a serious risk for sick people to attempt to solve medical problems without trained medical supervision. I may also mention that I have drawn information from reputable sources and have avoided ideas that are either controversial or in experimental state. However, I encourage readers to think for themselves and check the information rather than worshiping the ideas as a religion.

Maintaining health for mental and physical well-being, and delaying age-related damage to our body system involves different complex mechanisms. We can now control or partially control these mechanisms in our favor by proper health approaches. Our state of well-being or feeling good depends on the amount of energy available to us. The more energy available to our brain cells should make us feel brighter. The more energy available to all our cells should make us feel not only energetic, but also resistant to many diseases. For example, we know that people who are malnourished have a tremendously decreased resistance to diseases. In the last several years there has been an exciting development of interest in ways to help us avoid sickness, feel more energetic, and to live life to the fullest. Notable among these ways are the bioenergetics movement, transcendental meditation, group therapy, nutrition, breathing exercises, yoga and other exercise programs.

As you will realize, the main intention of this book is to utilize these programs for increasing the body's natural ability to produce more energy by following natural safe daily activities along with breathing exercises, yoga, and wholesome natural foods. These practical steps are not "gimmicks" but something that can be incorporated into a daily life style and stay with us for the rest of our lives. The degree of change to be felt will depend upon one's present health, as well as faith and closeness of following these habits.

If your health concerns are similar to an average person living in an affluent country such as the United States you have a fifty-fifty chance of dying of stroke or heart disease before your time. Our risk of getting arthritis, diabetes and cancer rises dramatically as we grow older. The hearing, eyesight, taste, smell, touch perceptions, all decline with age. In other words we slow down with age. This book can perhaps do something about these problems. It is intended not only to be read, but to be used actively. The real proof, of course, will lie within your own experience.

The overuse of drugs to treat everyday problems is another matter of serious concern. Drug use has become part of our daily living. In the United States alone over one billion dollars per year are spent on non-prescription drugs that are not needed. We buy drugs to help us sleep, cure our colds, and regulate our systems. We buy vitamins, cough remedies, dandruff cures and hair growers. We buy medications for upset stomachs, diarrhea, bad breath, athlete's foot, eczema, and headache. We do not try to understand the causes of above problems so that we can avoid the overuse of drugs, which may have bad effects on our health. Even the commonly used vitamin C in large doses may have serious side-effects. Large doses of vitamin C recommended by Professor Linus Pauling (Nobel Laureate in Chemistry) to prevent or cure a cold, may affect the kidneys, or even have bad effects on unborn infants during pregnancy. So, even though, vitamin C may help cure colds, it must be taken with care.

This book reminds you that good health is a natural state of the human body; and the natural healthy activities including wholesome natural foods, help in maintaining this state—and restoring it if it is lost—in ways that are natural to the body—not with powerful drugs. For example, carotenoids and retinoids (orange and yellow plant chemicals related to vitamin A) appear to offer important cancer prevention properties during the twenty-to-thirty-year lag phase in the development of human cancer, even after exposure has occurred. Japanese epidemiologists have shown that cigarette smokers who eat green and yellow vegetables have 30 per cent less cancer, compared to appropriately matched controls who do not eat these retinoid- and carotenoid-containing vegetables. A prudent diet that is low in fats and high in fresh fruits and vegetables is desirable, as is control over disease-provoking habits such as smoking, alcoholism and obesity.

In view of rising medical care costs, Ex-U.S. Secretary of Health and Human Resources (Richard Schweicker), has noted that prevention and more rational approaches to diseases and aging are mandatory. Approximately 100,000 coronary by-passes are performed yearly at an average cost of 50,000 each ($ 5 billion) and 1,000 people in U.S. alone die everyday of cancer. You see yourself that although we are making great advances in medical research and health technology and have increased an average life span, we see at the same time more people suffering from sickness. Many large hospital facilities are fully crowded with patients, and more medical insurance coverage is being purchased than ever before. I do not mean to ignore the medical achievements made in taming many of the killer diseases such as polio, tuberculosis and other infectious diseases, and advances in modern surgery. However, surgery should be needed only when preventable measures fail. For example, some of the heart operations can be avoided by putting patients on proper diet and exercise programs, as already being realized by some of the heart specialists in the United States.

It is important to note that health-related matters mentioned above, are not confined to a particular place, but to the entire world. We live in a global society within which it is possible for everyone to enjoy health, freedom, and happiness. We are now in a position to feed the hungry of the world with wholesome food which can provide economical sources of protein to keep people healthy—even in poor nations. To achieve these goals, we must begin with recovery of the physical and mental health of every person, family and community by the establishment of the wholesome health of each individual through the preventive practices. The need for medical care and facilities would become naturally reduced, except for some cases of emergencies.

It is with some of the above holistic ideas that *Health, Happiness, and Longevity* has been written, taking into consideration eastern as well as western thoughts and approaches. The use of this book could vary from individual readership of all age groups to general holistic health courses. It is practical enough to be read at a very straightforward level, yet it brings together information and philosophy to attract intellectual interest. With its potential for a broad appeal, this book belongs to every health-conscious person. This book is one of the most comprehensive books on holistic health that combines eastern and western approaches. However, you may be interested in one type of health area, a little interested in a few others, and not at all interested in the remainder. For those who feel that they have other things to do with their time than studying the entire book to understand the portion of their interest, the book is designed so that one does not have to read all of it. Each chapter contains a different topic. The chapters are further divided into headings and subheadings, so that one can quickly scan the contents of a chapter for a particular interest. Moreover, the quick scan of the entire book is made possible by summarizing the main points in a concluding Chapter 9. One can read the chapters of interest in an order different from the book. However, if you do not have background in nutrition, I recommend that you read Chapters 3 and 4 first, after which you can appreciate Chapter 5 on wholesome natural diet. The use of difficult scientific terms is minimized and these are often followed by a lay term in parentheses, e.g., lactose (milk sugar).

The information contained in the book came from innumerable sources such as reputable text books as well as popular best sellers by both eastern and western authorities, scientific journals, popular magazines (e.g., *Reader's Digest*), newspapers, television, and above all personal research and learning experiences. Several persons have helped in putting this book together.

I could never properly thank everyone who contributed to or influenced this work, but I would like to acknowledge a few very special people. To Dr. Laura Meagher, for stimulating discussions, for reading the manuscript, for constructive criticism, and for keeping my morale high, I am most appreciative. I am thankful to Mrs. Suzzane Sidhu and Mr. Nripinder Singh for reading the manuscript. I am also thankful to Professor Dr. Jerome Miksche, NCSU for reading Chapter 6 and for his discussions on eastern philosophy, and to Professor Dr. Graeme Berlyn, Yale University with whom, I had uncountable numbers of lunch discussions about health and life attitudes. Many thanks to the Department of Food Science, NCSU and my physician friends for helpful discussions that pertain to various parts of the book. I was always impressed by the interest and thoughtful discussions of my son Ameet Dhillon, who always believed in me and the book. Many thanks to my wife Rajvinder Dhillon for being understanding and for careful typing of the manuscript. Typing help was also provided by Mrs. Linda Stewart.

The picture credit goes to Mrs. Rosemary Stannett-Royce (last half of Chapter 8 pictures), Miss Gretchen Gjelhaug (first half of Chapter 8 pictures), Master Ameet Dhillon (Chapter 7 pictures), and the photographer Mr. Mark Edwards.

Last but not the least, I am grateful to Japan Publications, Inc. for their cooperation and understanding; it just pleased me to correspond with Mr. Iwao Yoshizaki and Mr. Yoshiro Fujiwara.

Contents

10

Introduction

Food, clothing, and shelter have been primary concerns of mankind for thousands of years. Over these years different cultures have developed various approaches to nutrition in several ways. When we look at eating patterns today, we can see diets that have been proven to work over centuries of experience, and diets which have been deliberately constructed over the past few years, based on fad, fancy, and oftentimes experimental evidence. Health-related scientific writings including the texts on nutrition by leading authorities such as Dr. Jean Mayer, formerly of Harvard Medical School, are informative in themselves and represent most of the information gained through laboratory experiments typical of scientific research. As a matter of fact, scientific experiments constitute one important way to collect accurate information. I may mention that as a scientist, I myself follow the same route and do trust the data collected from such experimentation. The particular information gained through these experiments is generally accurate, and therefore, diets based on these experiments may have many positive components. However, we cannot accept them as being conclusive. Diets constructed according to a particular set of specific data do not, and perhaps cannot, take into consideration all possible side effects or complications that may set in due to the inherently complex nature of biological systems. For example, the high protein diet fad took us away from carbohydrates which, along with fiber, are actually necessary to maintain good health and proper weight.

In contrast to the western experience, we have on the other hand, eastern notions on natural diet and yogic discipline which are based on centuries of experience but have not yet been fully subjected to experimental verification. As an analogy, the power of mind realized hundreds of years ago by yoga teachers is only recently being studied through a scientific approach by authorities in the field of hypnotism such as Dr. Spiegel of Columbia University. The ways in which experimental evidences are beginning to lend scientific support to common sense habits are perhaps the most interesting studies in the area of nutrition.

My western training as a scientist combined with perceptions of natural diet and yoga arising from my Indian heritage have been instrumental in the formation of the ideas that I have tried to develop here. The desire to explore any possible scientific bases for some common sense experiences was, in fact, the primary motivation for writing this manuscript. For example, as a young man growing up in the Punjab, India, I had heard that in the neighboring province of Rajsthan women had been using carrot seeds for a long time as a birth control measure. Today, this phenomenon is being studied scientifically at the All India Institute of Medical Sciences. Although no definite relationship between the seeds and their potential as fertility-controlling agents has yet been established, it has not been clearly disproved either. The knowledge of such instances has encouraged me to try to evaluate the scientific validity of natural diets.

The recent recommendations for reduced protein consumption, combined with high carbohydrate and fiber intake to achieve and maintain proper weight and good health are really nothing new. On examining common eating attitudes practiced in earlier societies we find that these had always been a part of their natural diet. Moreover, humans have biologically evolved with a natural diet, which simply includes wholesome foods in their natural state, primarily of plant origin; these are just the kind of foods with high carbohydrate and fiber that are associated with good health by recent scientific findings.

Unlike traditional writings on nutrition, this book places a special emphasis on nutritional evaluation of natural foods and their influence on our health. For instance, while methods of weight control range from fad diets to behavior modifications, the final answer to getting thin and staying thin seems to lie only in adopting a natural diet. Widespread adoption of this approach could save the United States alone over 10 billion dollars, the sum spent annually on weight reduction efforts (G. A. Bray. 1977. *Recent Advances in Obesity Research*. II. Newman Publishing, London. pp. 248–265). Vast as it is, the 10 billion dollar figure does not even include the medical costs resulting from the obesity-related diseases. Clearly, a weight problem exists in the United States, and equally clearly, much money and energy is directed towards it, often unsuccessfully. Thus there is room for a simple, straightforward approach to diet which depends on neither fads nor gimmicks, but on good common sense.

Natural diet foods can give sick people a new lease on life and save others from common diseases such as colon cancer and heart trouble. These foods can improve the vigor and vitality of those already in good health and contribute to their overall efficiency. We can go further and use the diet in prolonging life. This is treated in a separate chapter which includes the causes of aging and a safe practice of diet control to slow down the process in view of current aging theories.

This book is intended not only to provide a good understanding of nutrition and caloric values of food, and to explain explicitly the role of a natural diet in health, but also to foster a good general attitude towards healthy and happy living. Control over stress, and a healthy attitude towards everyday living are necessary prerequisites if the diet and health program is to work for you. Neither the diet nor the health program alone can be effective in prolonging life or making it healthier. Because books on either diet or health programs often fail to recognize this essential complementarity, many are unsatisfactory.

Taken in conjunction with nutrition and weight control discussed as the primary emphases of the book, simple rules to eliminate stress and a health program to energize the body are designed to help people of all ages to live longer, feel younger and lead a healthier life. In practicing the suggestions put forward in the pages of this book, the reader, it is hoped, will be able to enjoy a long disease-free life, full of health and happiness.

Chapter 1

A Healthy Attitude Towards a Happy Life

Everyone, whether saint or sinner, rich or poor, learned or ignorant, strives for happiness and not for misery. In other words, there is an inborn desire to be happy. Why is it then, that despite an instinctive desire to gain pleasure, people continue to experience unhappiness?

Struggle for Happiness

One of the foremost enemies of the happy life is the loss of initiative to be happy. Happiness is not always part of life, neither is it separated from life. Our traditional efforts to achieve happiness generally include materialistic living in search of physical comforts, seeking shelter in religious living or, in extreme cases, taking refuge in professional treatment and drugs. Professional treatment and drugs are clearly not a part of either happiness or hearlth, but are rather associated with sickness, i.e., health and happiness certainly exist outside the sick world of medicine and drugs. The approach of materialistic and selfish living oriented towards self-gain at the cost of hurting others also never leads to happiness in the long run. Such characters usually end up burning in the fire of their own selfish world. As far as religion is concerned, I agree that it has led many people twoards meaningful existence, but many others find it restrictive to the growth of a happy and healthy mind.

It may be interesting to note some of the findings about happiness, which support the above philosophy. These are concluded from a questionnaire, given to 52,000 people ranging in age from 15 to 95 (Shaver and Freedman, 1976, *Psychology Today*, p. 27).

1. Money can't buy happiness
2. Non-religious people are as happy as religious
3. Drugs, therapy, mysticism, or paranormal experiences don't bring happiness

Although many people prefer money because it provides freedom, true happiness exists in the head, not in the wallet. We must admit, of course that in the real world, people do need a certain amount of earnings, and it is easier to be happy if one is financially successful. However, the benefits of financial advantages generally do not last, and can be easily erased, for example, by overwork, stress, a bad home life, or a lack of motivation. Therefore those who use money as a vehicle towards happiness are highly unlikely to be successful. The race for money leaves some people hollow and dissatisfied. In fact, happiness has less to do with what you have than with what you want. It comes less often from absolute achievements than from relative ones.

As far as religion and happiness is concerned, religion in the broad sense may be helpful to certain people if it can teach them that life has meaning and direction. However, meaning and direction, important for adult happiness, may come more often from self-motivation. Religion, therefore, is not a prerequisite for happiness and non-religious people can be as happy as religious.

Drugs, therapy, mysticism or paranormal experiences are clearly an indication of sickness rather than happiness. These are often associated with emotional troubles during childhood or adulthood. In fact happiness is in the mind and for this reason, it is easy to criticize all the things which do not bring happiness. In the following pages we will turn our attention to the mind and attitudes which can be positively associated with happiness.

Happiness Comes from Tending Your Own Garden, Not Coveting Your Neighbor's

Happiness is a matter of setting personal standards, not chasing after other people's. Unfortunately, some people are so caught up in comparisons that they are unable to evaluate their own feelings. Happy people with proper attitudes are those who feel in control of their lives, and who compare their progress against their own standards, not those of others. Happiness has a lot to do with accepting and enjoying what one is and what one has, maintaining a balance between expectations and achievements.

A Few Suggestions for Healthy Attitudes

Suggestions for healthy attitudes towards happiness include:
1. Emotional security—believing that good things can last.
2. Belief that life has meaning, that one's guiding values are right.
3. Feeling of control over the things that happen, as opposed to feeling that one is merely a pawn of events.
4. Lack of cynicism—disagreeing that there is a sucker born every minute.

Health and happiness lie in leading a simple life while maintaining a healthy attitude composed of liveliness, fairness, helpfulness, sharedness. The important ingredients of happiness include (1) a kind heart which will not hurt even an enemy (2) a simple mind full of truth and sincerity (3) a healthy body which, with proper care, will allow us to carry on our healthy attitudes.

Caring for Your Body, a Healthy Step

Taking care of your body is a good indication of your healthy attitudes. Unfortunately, many individuals treat material goods better than their own bodies. Think of an object that you treasure very much—perhaps a work of art, a house, a garden, a car. Now concentrate on your own body; if you are like most people, you will realize that you treat your body less lovingly. The proper attitude toward health and happiness must start from paying attention and love to your body. If you have love and respect for your body, you would feel an integrated relationship between mind and body.

Good Habits, a Healthy Step

Our attitudes can be affected by our daily habits. Although our habits are considered our servants, they can also be devils and hurt us. That is why it is customary to call them good or bad habits. Over time, bad habits can be mentally as well as physically damaging.

A study by Lester Breslow, Dean, School of Public Health, UCLA, demonstrated that seven simple habits (listed below) can significantly determine a person's health status and life expectancy. An individual who practices all seven habits is expected to possess the health of a person thirty years younger than the one who ignores all of them. Life expectancy was correlated with the number of these habits which a person follows. For example, a forty-five-year-old person who practices three or less is likely to live to age sixty-seven, while a person of the same age who follows six or seven should live to seventy-eight (based on statistical correlations).

The followings are the seven simple habits that can add time and health to our lives.

1. Three regular meals a day, with few snacks
2. Breakfast regularly
3. Moderate exercise two or three times a week
4. Moderate weight
5. Seven to eight hours sleep a night (not more)
6. No smoking
7. Little or no alcohol

According to Dean Breslow's results, most people surveyed averaged two or three of these habits. I agree that it is not easy to break a habit, but with self-determination and faith in what is said in the pages of this book, it is quite possible to break old habits, routines, and behavior that interfere with your health. For example, when you take an aspirin to cure a headache, try to understand the source or stressful situation which caused it. Taking aspirin only suppresses the headache temporarily; the permanent cure is to treat the cause of the headache.

Many psychotherapists suggest programs like the one below to develop healthful habits or to change into a healthful one. The main steps of the program may be briefly listed in the following sequential stages:

1. Observe yourself to discover exactly the nature of the habit and the circumstances under which it evolved. For example, see if your headache follows after doing something you dislike or by meeting someone who upsets you. Only after understanding the cause, you can find a solution to avoid the situation.
2. Motivation or willpower is the next step to change the habit after you become aware of the problem. For example, sugar, tobacco, or alcohol

consumption would be reduced, if these were illegal; the same can be achieved by willpower.

3. Design a program to change a habit. For example, to lose weight decide the weight to be lost (say 35 pounds) and time (say 6 months), and adopt an eating and exercising program to achieve it.

4. The fourth step of the program involves adopting new and healthier habits. New habits, although at first they may seem unnatural, become automatic and easy after practice. For example, you can get used to waking up early in the morning after a few weeks of inconvenience.

5. Controlling your environment is another step towards learning new responses. For example, if you are trying to quit smoking, it is helpful if your family and friends do not smoke.

These suggestions may not offer a miraculous program, but they can lead you to control over damaging habits. The unhealthy habits can change, if you understand their roots, and restructure the environment to create incentives for new habits.

Self-Affirmation, a Healthy Step

Constructive assessment of your mistakes and short-comings is a healthy attitude, but calling yourself names, or expressing frustration at your limitations can create a negative emotional effect on your body. The latter can easily lead to self-punishment and self-hate, which can end up in psychic pain, worry, depression, anxiety or physical illness. By contrast, repeating positive, self-affirming suggestions to yourself as discussed in next Chapter 2, can help mobilize your expectant faith in your future and your inner potential for self-health and happiness.

In many spiritual and healing traditions, as well as in praying, the power of positive mental images has been a major source of healing for healthful living. Today these old traditions are supported by scientific findings which demonstrate conclusively the effect of mind over body. Science has provided technical interpretations for what was formerly explained as divine intervention.

Below are some points of positive-image meditation. Notice that all of these phrases are in the present tense, proclaiming that they are happening now. There is no wishing or hoping involved.

1. Every day in every way I am getting better and better, becoming more alive and healthy
2. My mind is quiet, still and happy
3. My body is calm and relaxed
4. I am one with all living things
5. I accept myself completely
6. I am filled with energy
7. I am letting go of my unrealistic expectations about my work and family
8. I use my consciousness to be free of outside forces
9. I have everything within myself to enjoy every minute of every day

Although the above points about positive images may seem simple and childish, you may be surprised at their power to lead you towards healthy attitudes. These can help you to remake your future—first in your imagination and then in actuality.

Joy of Self—Eastern Philosophy

As mentioned earlier, the happiness is in mind. However, when one tries to relax the mind, one cannot completely remove all tensions and worries from the mind unless one goes to spiritual relaxation. There is no way of obtaining complete relaxation and happiness, unless one can withdraw himself from the body idea and separate himself from the ego consciousness. By withdrawing himself, one identifies himself with the all-pervading, all-powerful, all-peaceful and joyful self or pure consciousness within himself. Knowledge of self, which destroys ignorance, provides direct means to liberation. However, man's quest for knowledge will never be complete until he turns his wisdom inward. The *Upanishads* declare that all knowledge is in the self. In addition to attaining the knowledge, every man is made to exist and to have a joyous nature; this triple nature of the self is known as *sat-chit-ananda* (existence, knowledge, and bliss).

According to Eastern philosophy, the quest for happiness goes on endlessly because people are vainly searching for something that they seem to have lost. That something is the joy of the self or soul which exists within them. Unfortunately, they seek it outside the self. Take, for example, a person who has all the material possessions he can ever desire. But does he have complete happiness? Not likely, for material desires multiply. No sooner has a person made his first million than he would desire four. This goes on endlessly. Now, why does one feel unsatisfied even after acquiring all the worldly possessions that he desires? The primary sources of dissatisfaction or even misery is the sense of "I-ness" and "mineness." For example, a man experiences extreme sorrow at the loss of wife, son, or wealth, but not at the loss of an enemy, because in the later case there is no "I-ness" or "mineness" involved. The joyous nature of the self gets clouded with what we call love or attraction for gross bodies and external things. Just as effort is made to diminish "I-ness" and "mineness," pain and sorrow vanish, because sorrow is not an inherent property of a person. The realization of self or soul, therefore, is the more appropriate goal to strive for. Even a little knowledge of the self brings great joy and courage to those afflicted by pain and miseries of the world. Though the absolute realization of the self for ordinary people at the present state of evolution may take a long time, one could get great joy and comfort by following the plain ideas advanced in this book while doing his worldly duties.

Chapter 2

Full Living

We cannot spend our lives in dream or fantasy; the need to deal with the real world is too overwhelming. However, our fantasies do certainly exist in some corner of reality. That corner is precisely the place where our happiness is hiding. Enthusiasm is the first step in finding that hidden spot. Life is a balance between enthusiasm and inhibition. If enthusiasm dominates inhibition, life can be full of liveliness and satisfaction, but if inhibition dominates, life will be empty. An over-enthusiastic personality can sometimes hurt itself, but it is certainly better than an empty life dominated by inhibition. In the long run, it is the enthusiast who finds the happy corner of life, because his enthusiastic mind cannot let itself be occupied with inhibited and miserable feelings. Enthusiasm is not always a part of life, but it can be created by efforts. Whenever feelings of inhibition occupy the mind, efforts should be made to kick out the inhibitory feelings to make a place for enthusiasm. The people we call lucky are the ones full of enthusiasm. They are the soul of the world. Happiness and success depends on a healthy, enthusiastic mind.

Although enthusiasm can lead you to a full living, you cannot avoid completely the ups and downs of a real life. The suggestions below can be very helpful in facing everyday life situations.

A Few Western and Eastern Suggestions to Face Everyday Situations

Full and happy living needs a free mind which should be in close contact with soul and body. Body, soul and mind are the doors to a happy life. The simple suggestions below, the desiderata stemming from the Western tradition, can be helpful in keeping mind, body, and soul in harmony with each other. Some of these may already be familiar to you, as they have recently achieved popularity in the U.S.

1. Go placidly amid the noise and haste, and think what peace there may be in silence.
2. As far as possible, without surrender, be on good terms with all persons. Speak your truth quietly and clearly; and listen to others, even the dull and ignorant. They too have their story.
3. Avoid loud and aggressive persons, they are vexatious to the spirit.
4. If you compare yourself with others, you may become vain and bitter; for always there will be greater and lesser persons than yourself.
5. Enjoy your achievements as well as your plans.

6. Keep interested in your own career, however humble; it is a real possession in the changing fortunes of time.

7. Be yourself. Especially do not feign affection. Neither be cynical about love; for in the face of all aridity and disenchantment it is perennial as the grass.

8. You are a child of the universe, no less than the trees and the stars; you have a right to be here. Therefore be at peace with God, whatever you conceive him to be, and whatever the labors and aspirations, in the noisy confusion of life keep peace with your soul.

9. With all its sham, drudgery and broken dreams, it is still a beautiful world. Be careful. Strive to be happy.

The following suggestions emerging from Eastern philosophy supplement the ideas stated above:

1. Remember that worry, anxiety and fear will not solve any problem. If there is a problem, collect the facts, then ask yourself what is the worst possible result that can happen, and decide to accept even this if necessary. Dismiss the problem from your mind but maintain hope and the expectation of a good result.

2. Have a goal which you can hope to attain. If it is too high it will result in discouragement if you fail. When you succeed, then raise the standard, step by step.

3. Be temperate in all things. Avoid extremes. Take a more detached view of life, neither over-elated by success nor depressed by failure.

4. Think before you act. A wrong thought can be rectified more quickly than a wrong action. When questioned, think and then reply; try not to jump to conclusions, have a positive attitude to everything you do or think about. Negative attitudes invite failure.

5. Have a plan for each day, but do not be a slave to the plan.

6. When concentrating your thought on a problem, give particular attention to relaxing the muscles round the forehead, eyes and mouth.

7. Think about other people rather than about yourself. Do not be a cause of injury to others. Be compassionate. Forgive the weaknesses of others.

8. Learn to withdraw into an inner privacy of mind even in the thickest crowd.

Stress and Full Living

One of the common interferences in the enjoyment of living today are the experiences of stress, anxiety and tension. The obvious effects of such experiences are: an increase in pulse rate and an increased tendency to sweat; one generally becomes more irritable and oftentimes suffer insomnia; one generally becomes less capable of concentrating and has an increased desire to move about; one feels muscle tensing in the neck and shoulders and develops a headache; one can have an upset stomach and indigestion along with change in appetite; one feels exhaustion and decreased desire for sex; many times there is also an excessive feeling of guilt. All the demands one makes—whether on the brain or the liver or the muscles or the bones—cause stress, which can be defined as the nonspecific response of the body to any demand. Most people who are ambitious and want to accomplish something, however, live on some stress as a part of regular living. They need it. In other words, accomplishment requires work, and the regular work, which is an essential part of full living itself causes some stress.

Dr. Hans Selye, the acknowledged authority on stress writes that our aim should not be to avoid work but to find the kind of work that suits us best. The best way to avoid undue stress is to select an environment (wife, husband, boss, social group) in line with our innate preferences, and an activity which we like and respect and which is within our talents. In this way we can eliminate the need for constant adaptation which is the major cause of harmful stress. Hard workers in almost any field often live to a very advanced age. A common example which supports the above notions is that employed wives are, generally, happier than housewives.

So far we have learnt that we can't live without some stress to enjoy full living, and even to strive for happiness itself implies some stress. However, too much stress can literally kill us. Many times the effects of stress are not dramatic and people continue to function without becoming aware of its effects. It makes them irritable, and unnecessarily critical of their friends, family or co-workers. It may cause people to overreact to little annoyances; and may cause other symptoms such as decreased desire for sex. However, excessive exposure to stress over a long time may cause serious diseases such as hypertension, heart accidents, nervous disorders. The treatment of stress in such cases is an absolute necessity.

Unfortunately, if you were to ask a typical physician for relief from stress, he would probably prescribe tranquilizers. The most widely prescribed and abused tranquilizer is Valium, which has nerve calming and muscle relaxing ingredients. The sales for Valium in 1979 were over $130 million. Although Valium and other similar drugs may be of value in the treatment of anxiety and tension associated with situational states, drug dependency and side effects are serious problems. These pills decrease a person's awareness of stress, producing the "tranquilizing" effect, but they have no effect on the autonomic nervous system, the arousal state, or the stress response by which the body reacts to tension. Thus, relief from pills is only temporary unless the stress- or anxiety-producing situation in the environment is changed. The tranquilizers only mask the properties of stress and are not a means to true relaxation at all. Many non-medical alternatives to stress relief, such as alcohol and tobacco, do the same, covering up stress rather than reversing or curing it.

Among natural ways to relax, the most familiar to us is sleep. In addition to providing rest, dreaming during sleep eliminates the day's tensions in some incompletely understood-way. Sleeping pills decrease the ability to dream, thus blocking the natural stress-relieving mechanism. The use of sleeping pills, therefore, can result in an accumulation of the harmful effects of stress. Another natural way which can provide some relief from stress is physical exercise. However, the progressive ways to provide relief from stress are mental approaches based on ancient methods, some of which are supported by scientific research.

The Role of the Mind in Controlling Stress and Improving Life

Many people who are called meditators allow their mind to experience a relaxed and enjoyable state which draws their attention inward. Our average daily experience consists of an unending cascade of thoughts, emotions, sensations and perceptions. The disengagement from these continuous impressions allows the attention to shift inward to experience quiet levels of the mind. Regular practice of such experiences leads to relief from stress. Similar relief can come from the discipline of body and mind through the practice of breathing, yoga, walking and healthful nutrition as discussed in the later chapters. The physiology of advanced practitioners of yoga and breathing exercises has shown similarities to the physiology of practitioners of transcendental meditation (Bloomfield, Cain and Jaffe. *TM*. Delacorte Press, NY, 1975). Clinical experiments on people who use mental approaches such as meditation to relieve stress have supported such claims as slow pulse rate and oxygen consumption, decreased anxiety, and increased concentration. Therefore the practice of transcendental meditation along with yogic discipline and breathing exercises should be the most effective way to improve physical as well as mental well being.

Meditation in simple words can be defined as a state of mind when unpleasant thoughts are blocked and concentration is focused on some pleasant thought or a word which is called a *mantra*, e.g. the word 'OM.' However, the claim is often made that the mantra must be taught by a trained teacher of meditation and it can never be learned from a book. For this reason, one of the popular books on transcendental meditation by Bloomfield, Cain and Jaffe (*TM*. Delacorte Press, NY, 1975) explains all about meditation and its benefits but leaves the reader with no specific suggestions other than to look for a meditation center (a list of centers in the United States is provided). There is absolutely no practical information that can allow a reader to utilize the mental approach of relaxation such as meditation to improve the quality of life.

Like most people, you probably need a practical program rather than philosophy to relax tight muscles and to decrease worry and anxiety. The exercises in the following pages, including a meditation approach, suggest wakeful relaxation procedures to enable you to deal actively with the stress response. Many of these can be practiced successfully by yourself without the need of a center or a Guru or a teacher.

Methods of Relaxation Based on Mental Approaches

All mental approaches to relaxation—including meditation and autogenic training—are technically forms of self-hypnosis. Using these techniques, a person talks directly to his unconscious mind, suggesting a state of relaxation. The learning of these relaxation techniques is not too difficult, but the commitment is the difficult task. While some people experience an immediate positive impact, others do not feel any initial benefits. However, even for the latter, change will come with time. Hopefully, one day either physicians will prescribe or patients will learn to attend relaxation classes, rather than using a tranquilizer such as Valium, for chronic stress.

To practice relaxation use a "passive attention" approach, i.e., relax not by forcing yourself to, but simply allowing it to happen. Passive attention is difficult to describe and it must really be experienced to be fully understood. If you give yourself a command, or concentrate or try too hard, you will achieve the results opposite to the one you desire. A few people initially experience the relaxation exercise as causing more tension rather than less. Despite what you may encounter, it is important to continue practicing the exercise. Try the exercises given below. You will probably feel comfortable with at least one of them, and that is the one you can regularly use.

Progressive Relaxation: Get into a comfortable position, such as the meditative position or yoga relaxation posture given in Chapter 8. You may want to lie down on a bed or a rug, or sit in a chair. If you tend to fall asleep, sitting up or one of the meditative positions is better.

When you are comfortable, transfer your awareness from the outside world to inside your body. To do this, close your eyes, and become aware of your breathing. Breathing is the source of life energy (as emphasized in Chapter 7), and the connection between your inner world and outer world. You may focus on your breath moving into your mouth, down your windpipe, and into your lungs, and perhaps imagine even down into your stomach and solar plexus, and then out again, into the world. Spend a few minutes inhaling deeply and exhaling slowly. Let your breathing be effortless and spontaneous. Let it happen by itself without consciously forcing it. Whenever your mind begins to wander, simply return your awareness to your breathing, but don't get upset, don't try to fight it.

After regulating your breath and pausing for a few minutes, now become sensitive to your entire body. Beginning at the top of your head, place your awareness in each part of your body. How does it feel and look for your mind's eye to be in the top of your head? Are you aware of any tension or discomfort there? If so, simply breathe into that area. Imagine your breath going there and cleansing and bathing it with energy. As you exhale, imagine passing all the tension or discomfort out of that part of your body, and also notice the feeling of heaviness in that part of the body. Continue to breathe deeply and slowly.

Now let your consciousness descend to your face. How does it feel? Is there any tension or discomfort? If so, let your breath bathe that area, and as you exhale, release the tension in your face. Experience how pleasurable and relaxed your face now feels.

Then do the same with each part of your body: first your neck, then your shoulders, your arms (one by one), your hands, chest, stomach, waist, genitals, hips, legs, feet. When you focus your attention on each part, let the air flow in and bathe that area, soothing it, and releasing any tension. Then experience the pleasure of that part of your body being relaxed.

Spend a few minutes enjoying your relaxed body, and the calm feelings that are now part of it. Become aware of your breathing once more, and with each exhalation, feel the last little bit of tension leaving your body. Notice the pleasant feelings as you exhale. Continue for a few more minutes. Then, slowly return your awareness to the room.

Try to prolong the sensation of well-being, relaxation, and peacefulness as you return to your activities for the day. Whenever you are under stress, you can simply sit down and recall this state of relaxation, and from memory, you will be able to recreate it at will.

The first few times you perform this exercise, spend a full half hour scanning your body and releasing tension. Eventually, with practice you will learn to move through your body in less than 10 minutes, releasing tensions wherever they exist. Some people find it difficult to learn to do this without some help. One easy and convenient way is to make a tape recording of the relaxation procedure in a calm, leisurely voice and then play it back, following along.

Self-Hypnosis/Mental Relaxation: As described for the preceding exercise, get into a comfortable position, either sitting or lying down. Focus your eyes intently on a spot directly ahead of you, until your eyes feel tired and your vision begins to blur, then roll your eyeballs to the top of your head and shut your eyelids. Imagine you feel a warm cloud bathing the center of your body. As the cloud touches you, it will warm and relax that part of your body.

Next imagine that the cloud is slowly expanding from your center, growing larger, and touching each part of your body in turn with its warmth, energy, and peace. You are totally bathed in the revitalizing cloud, which releases any tension within you.

When you are entirely engulfed in the cloud, feel your body become lighter, warmer, and calmer. Imagine yourself beginning to float upward, completely weightless, soaring into the sky. The cloud with you at the center, takes you to a special place, where you can be completely calm, relaxed, and at peace. Visualize how beautiful that place is. Imagine how it looks, smells, sounds, and tastes. Also recognize how pleasant you feel in there, how vital, warm, alert, relaxed, healthy, and calm you are. Experience the pleasure of total well-being.

When you decide to return your awareness to the room, simply imagine yourself descending once again on the cloud and being settled gently back in your room. Before you open your eyes and complete your return, however, spend a moment recalling how you felt, and remind yourself that you can reexperience that sensation anytime you wish. Take some of that feeling of peace and well-being with you for the rest of your day. When you are ready, open your eyes, and sit quietly for a few moments.

Autogenic Training: Autogenic training is a series of messages, called orientations. During the training a person suggests or imagines these orientations to himself while sitting in a comfortable, relaxed state. These messages activate a visceral response, which deepens relaxation. Autogenic training generally requires a longer training period than that of progressive relaxation. If faithfully done, however, it will reinforce your ability to relax at will.

To begin a modified form of autogenic exercise, lie comfortably on your back, or on a recliner chair, and repeat the phrase "I am at peace." Say it slowly, again and again, for about a minute. Do not force yourself to concentrate on it, and if you find your mind drifting, gently bring yourself back to it. After a minute of practice, rest and then repeat the same process again. Continue alternating between rest and focusing several more times.

After you have practiced this initial phrase, you are ready to coordinate with breathing. As you breathe in, begin to imagine, or think, or repeat to yourself, the phrase "I am," and as you breathe out, repeat to yourself the phrase "at peace." This is your personal meditation mantra that you can use to begin to suggest the feeling of peace, warmth, and well-being throughout your body. Just pay attention to your breathing: inhaling "I am," exhaling "at peace." Feel your body respond, "I am—at peace."

After you have practiced the initial phrase, use a series of suggestions or commands to your body. They will induce a deep, calm, restful state of activation of the parasympathetic nervous system. The basic suggestions or orientations are: (1) my right arm is heavy (2) my right hand is warm (3) my pulse is calm and regular (4) my abdomen is warm (5) my forehead is pleasantly cool.

Now to perform the exercise, concentrate on your right arm. Pay attention only to your right arm and then say to yourself, "My right arm is heavy." Repeat this for about 90 seconds, three times a day, over a period of two weeks. Once you have a feeling of restful heaviness in the right arm. Say: "My right arm is heavy, my left arm is heavy; both arms are heavy," and again repeat the total procedure three times a day. Then one leg then the other leg and then both legs are added. Then combine with the phrase my hands are warm.

Next concentrate on making both your arms and legs heavy and hands warm. Following the development of warmth, you concentrate on making your heart beat calmly and regularly, saying, for example my pulse is calm and regular. Finally, concentrate on a feeling of warmth in the abdomen and a feeling of coolness in the forehead. After, say, six months of this progressive training, most individuals are able to relax each part of the body quickly and totally at any given moment.

Transcendental Meditation: As with any other mental approach to relaxation, the ultimate goal of meditation is to make contact with the unconscious and allow its wisdom to guide you in the relaxing process. Our average daily experiences are full of countless inner forms, thoughts, feelings, memories, and ideas which are with us, even if we are physically shut off from the outer world by sitting in an isolated area. Meditation is the process which helps to break this chain of random thoughts and impressions by allowing us to learn to do one thing at a time. By concentrating on a single thing—whether it be your breath, your garden, or your jogging—you will enter not only an altered state of consciousness, but also an altered (and more positive) state of physiology.

To begin meditation, find a quiet place free of distractions. Because you want your mind to get into the habit of regularly attaining a state of meditation, it is better to create a regular time and location for your daily meditation. It should generally not take place immediately after a meal. A meditation site becomes so special for many people that they decorate it with personal or symbolic objects to affirm its significance. Such gestures indicate the seriousness of commitment to the process.

To practice the meditation exercise, sit quietly in a position where your back is straight (e.g. one of meditation positions given in Chapter 8), supported, if need be, by the back of the chair. Close your eyes.

Make a quick inventory of your body, checking for any special tensions or discomforts. Become aware of any tightness, tension, or strain in your muscles. If you find some tension, breathe in and then, on exhalation, gently but firmly relax your muscles as much as possible.

When your physical evaluation is completed, you should perform a mental and emotional inventory. If you find any special anxiety or uncomfortable thought, experience it for a few moments, but then ease it out of your mind. Rather than trying to force it away, simply allow the thought to flow out of your awareness by turning your attention away from it. You may not be able to remove yourself entirely from your concerns, but at least this method provides a start.

You should now be relaxed both physically and mentally. Begin breathing, without forcing your attention to it. That is, utilize passive volition rather than active concentration. Instead of attempting to coerce away thoughts that distract you from your breathing, let them come. When you become aware of them, consciously return all your attention to your breathing. Do not expect your mind to remain easily focused on your breathing. During a ten-to-twenty-minute meditation, you can anticipate that your mind will wander away many times. But be patient. You are still meditating well, even if your mind does wander. The meditation process consists of bringing your mind back, time after time, to your breathing, until focused attention becomes a habit. Rather than just centering on your breathing, you may find it easier to count breaths. As you inhale, silently count "one." In the exhalation, say "and." The next breath is "two," and so on, until you get to "four," when you begin again. If you lose count, start again at "one."

As you concentrate on your breathing—whether by visualizing, counting, or any other method—do not try to alter or control it in any way. Instead, let your breathing regulate itself, spontaneously and effortlessly.

About ten to twenty minutes after beginning this exercise, you should be ready to conclude it. Stop concentrating on your breathing. This will return you to your normal stream of awareness. Blink your eyes several times, then open them and sit quietly for a minute or two. When you get up, you will feel refreshed and energized.

There is a great range of initial responses to this meditation exercise. Some people feel peaceful and relaxed immediately. Others sense very little change at first and have almost had to restrain themselves from stopping the exercise by jumping from their seats. Still others, although determined to make the exercise work, discover themselves replaying worries or problems they have, finding it impossible to still these thoughts.

However, it may be reassuring simply to know that these problems are common. People usually begin relaxation or meditation with many positive preconceptions and expectations, and when they don't materialize—when the mind isn't instantly still, or it continues to think the same thoughts it did at other times of the day— they see themselves as failures. But skill at relaxation cannot be bought ready- made; it must be gradually developed. Even when it seems you are not making any progress, the exercise is probably having some beneficial effects.

A Simplified Method of Mind Relaxation for Sleep: As we mentioned earlier, meditation suggests blocking thoughts about the day's worries and concentrating on a pleasant thought or simple word called a mantra, the most popular being "OM." The following relaxation exercise should be very helpful for inducing sleep. At the time of sleeping, as you lie down on the bed, stretch your body and legs, relaxing every possible muscle. Lie in any comfortable position which suits you. You can lie with face upward, to the right or to the left. Now, after relaxing your body, concentrate on any word which will not bother you and which you can associate with faithfully. "OM" may be used or any other word or scene or favorite music or experience about nature, love, and so on, that you choose. You may even concentrate on your own body parts, concentrating on and mentally relaxing each body part from toes to head as given in the relaxation posture of yoga in Chapter 8. After choosing a focus of attention, concentrate and repeat or visualize it repeatedly so that no other thought can occupy your mind. If done properly, you should fall asleep in few minutes in a very relaxed state. Do the same in the morning just after you wake up. Then stretch your body while prone to activate energy. After a few minutes from the time of waking up, you will be fresh and willing to get out of bed for the day's activities.

Both the length of time and the way we sleep ultimately affect our personalities and our physiological well-being. Extreme changes in sleep habits, from the nor- mal 7 to 8 hours, could be symptomatic of changes in emotional and/or physio- logical health. The best position for sleep is either on the back or the side. When people sleep on their stomachs, the weight of the body prevents the diaphragm and the rib cage from properly expanding; this interferes with deep diaphragmatic breathing (see Chapter 7).

The relaxation exercises mentioned above may not solve all emotional prob- lems, but they are a very useful tool to face the strains of life. They can help us to control our bodies and minds and to function more effectively and more con- structively. They can reduce the beating our bodies take as they react to the pulls and pushes of jobs, families and crises.

Chapter **3**

Nutrition and Nutrients

The process by which living organisms receive and utilize food is known as
nutrition; and the life-sustaining constituents in food are called *nutrients*. During
an average life time of 70 years, a person who at any time weighs no more than
165 pounds eats 35 tons of food, the equivalent of 16,000 bricks or enough to build
two three-bedroomed houses. Clearly, there is a need to learn about food, which
is consumed in such a large quantity. Most people develop eating habits early in
life that are in accord with social and family patterns, and modify them only
slightly over the years. Sometimes these habits conform to ideal food recommendations from the viewpoint of maintaining and fostering good health. More
often, however, they do not. Gaining knowledge about food and its relationship
to health is the best way to change inappropriate eating patterns of adults and to
introduce youngsters to good eating habits that should last a life time. Therefore,
everyone needs to learn a few facts about food and health as a basis for selecting
the foods to eat.

Moreover, to understand and evaluate for yourself the suggested natural diet
(Chapter 5), basic knowledge about nutrients and their role in our diet is important. With this knowledge, it is likely that you would find a natural diet to be the
best for health in general, and for weight control, elimination of certain diseases
and longevity in particular.

Food is required for two basic reasons which are very important to understand
in maintaining health and controlling weight.

1. Food provides the nutrients that are essential for the building, the upkeep,
    and the repair of body tissues as well as those required for the efficient
    functioning of the body.
2. Food gives energy for work and play, to move, to breathe, to keep the
    heart beating, just to be alive. For children and youth food provides energy
    to support growth.

Nutrients and Their Functions

The 50 or so known nutrients needed for proper functioning of the body include
proteins (amino acids), carbohydrates (sugar and starches), fats (fatty acids),
minerals, vitamins, and water (Table 3.1). These nutrients are widely distributed
in our foods yet no single food, not even milk, meat or eggs, contains all the
nutrients.

Proteins and Essential Amino Acids: From the smallest virus to the largest whale, all life requires protein for existence. This is so because much of the body's structure is made up of proteins. For example, a typical 150-pound person is composed of about 94 pounds of water, 27 pounds of protein, 23 pounds of fat, 5 pounds of minerals (mostly in bones), 1 pound of carbohydrates, and less than an ounce of vitamins. If we exclude water, about 50 percent of the body weight is protein, which is comprised of hundreds of different kinds of proteins, each with special properties and functions. Skin, hair, nails, muscles, cartilage tendons, blood, and even the organic framework of bones are made up largely of proteins. Most of the protein is found in muscle tissue; the remainder is distributed in soft tissues, bones, teeth, blood and other body fluids.

Table 3.1 The major classes of nutrients, their main functions and food sources.

Nutrient	Functions	Main Food Sources
Proteins	Build, repair tissue Regulate body processes Supply energy Fight infection	Meat, fish, poultry, dried beans, peas, seeds, nuts, cheese, eggs, cereal grains
Carbohydrates	Supply energy Spare protein Aid in burning of fat Provide fiber	Grains, fruits, vegetables, milk
Fats	Provide the essential fatty acid, linoleic acid Promotes absorption of fat-soluble vitamins A, D, E, K Supply energy	Fats and oils, nuts, meat, fish, poultry, dairy products, some seeds
Minerals	Regulate body processes Maintain body tissues	All foods except sugar, alcohol and refined fats and oils
Vitamins	Regulate body processes Maintain tissue structure and function	All foods except sugar, alcohol and refined fats and oils
Water	Transport nutrients Regulates body temperature Participates in chemical reactions Removes waste material	Water, beverages, and almost all foods have some water

Chemically, the protein is made up of smaller units called amino acids which contain various elements such as carbon, hydrogen, oxygen, nitrogen and sometimes sulfur. The protein we eat from various food sources is not used as such, but is broken down into amino acids in the digestive tract and then absorbed into the blood stream. These amino acids travel in the blood to all parts of the body wherever cells need them. In tissues throughout the body, the amino acids are then rearranged to form many special and distinct proteins. The rearrangement of amino acids to produce the long-chain polymers that we call proteins may be regarded as a reaction between amino acids in which water molecules are eliminated. After elimination of water, the remaining protein of the two amino acids thus become linked by a chemical grouping called a peptide bond. The number of amino acids linked to form a chain of protein may vary from as small as 23 to as large as several hundred thousand amino acid units. The order or sequence in which amino acids are linked is determined by genetic make up of an individual, stored in the DNA molecule (DNA is the material from which genes are made). It is DNA which determines the different types of proteins such as blond hair protein or black hair protein.

Table 3.2   Classification of amino acids required for body's protein needs.

Essential (need to be supplied as formed molecules)	Nonessential (can be synthesized from cellular substances)
Isoleucine	Alanine
Leucine	Asparagine
Lysine	Aspartic Acid
Methionine	Citrulline
Phenylalanine	Cystine
Threonine	Glutamic acid
Tryptophan	Glutamine
Valine	Glycine
Arginine*	Hydroxyproline
Histidine*	Proline
	Serine
	Tyrosine

* Essential only for the growing child.

There are 22 different amino acids that are required for the body's protein needs (Table 3.2). Eight of these must come ready-made from food and are called essential amino acids; the rest can be synthesized by the body itself and are termed nonessential. This is not to suggest that the nonessential amino acids are not essential constituents of the protein, but rather that the tissue can make their own supply from carbohydrate, fat and other amino acids. An important requirement for the synthesis of a protein is the simultaneous availability of all the amino acids needed for a particular protein. This is so, because protein synthesis is not a step-wise process. Complete peptides are laid down in a short period of time and there is no provision for storage of incomplete sections. Even the temporary unavailability of single essential amino acid can interfere with protein synthesis and stop it altogether. Knowledge about the nutritional value of foods is, therefore, important to ensure the supply of all the necessary amino acids.

Proteins from animal origin such as meat, fish, poultry, eggs, and milk supply all of the necessary amino acids. Proteins from cereal grains, vegetables, and fruits also supply valuable amounts of many amino acids. As discussed in detail in Chapter 5, a vegetarian person can stay as healthy as a non-vegetarian by using plenty of legumes such as soybeans and chickpeas in the diet along with milk to supply essential amino acids, some of which are found only in animal proteins. The minimum requirement of essential amino acids for an adult is readily obtained in four slices of bread and one pint of milk. Similarly, cereal and milk, or macaroni and cheese, form good combinations to provide the essential amino acids (see Chapter 5 for details of food combinations).

The proteins are needed all through life for the maintenance and repair of body tissues. Children urgently need proteins for normal growth, and adults need it for continually growing tissue such as hair and nails. The protein in hair, skin, and nails is hard and insoluble, providing a protective coating for the body. The protein of muscle allows this tissue to contract and hold water. The elastic protein of blood vessels allow them to expand and contract to maintain normal blood pressure. Protein also provides the rigid frame work for the minerals of bones and teeth. The building of cells is only one of the roles of protein in the body. Among other functions, proteins help to (1) make hemoglobin, the blood protein that carries oxygen to the cells and carries carbon dioxide away from the cells (2) form antibodies that fight infection and combat foreign invaders like disease-causing bacteria (3) supply energy to the body (4) hormones—such as insulin and adrenaline that regulate certain body functions—are also protein in nature.

Carbohydrates: Foods supply carbohydrates chiefly in three forms—starches, sugars, and celluloses. Celluloses along with hemicelluloses, lignin, pectin and cutin, furnish fibrous bulk in the diet. These complex compounds are substances found in the cell walls of various plants and quantity of each substance depends on the specific plant and may vary with each species. It has been suggested that fiber may play a role in preventing cancer and diseases of the intestinal tract, lowering blood cholesterol and promoting weight loss as discussed in detail in Chapter 5. The most familiar forms of carbohydrates, starches and sugars, are the major sources of energy for humans and must be available in the body constantly. It takes about 2 pounds of carbohydrates to provide a 160-pound person with fuel for the whole day. In the absence of a carbohydrate supply, body fat and protein will be converted to sugar for energy supply, a potentially dangerous situation (see section "Fad Diets" in Chapter 4). Unless there is an excess of body fat, it is not desirable to go without a carbohydrate supply. In any event, once the stored supply of fat is used up, the need for carbohydrates becomes imperative.

All carbohydrates are readily broken down by digestive enzymes into their component sugars and absorbed into the blood stream. Glucose, commonly called blood sugar, is the form in which starches and sugars are mainly used by cells to furnish energy. Except for milk and milk products, which contain the sugar lactose, nearly all the carbohydrates we eat originally come from plants. Good sources of carbohydrates are grains, fruits, and vegetables. The health risks of using excessive refined carbohydrates such as sugar are discussed later in this chapter in a section on controversial chemicals.

Fats: Fats are chemically complex food components composed of glycerol and fatty acids. Fats are commonly classified as saturated and unsaturated, which simply denote saturation and unsaturation of the molecular structure by hydrogen atoms. The saturated fats are suggested to increase the cholesterol content of the blood, whereas the unsaturated fats found in fish and vegetable oil do not add to the blood cholesterol content. In choosing daily meals, it is good to keep the total amount of fat at a moderate level and to include some foods that contain unsaturated fats.

Fats play several essential roles in the metabolic process. As concentrated sources of energy (270 calories per ounce), they provide more than twice as much energy, or calories, as either carbohydrates or protein. Therefore, body fats are an efficient way to store energy, and also an easy way to accumulate excess calories in a diet. The body uses these stored calories when it needs more energy than the diet supplies. That's why one loses body fat on a low-calorie diet. Fats serve as carriers of the fatsoluble vitamins A, D, E, and K. Fats also make up part of the structure of cells, form a protective cushion around vital organs, insulate the body against cold temperature, and supply an essential fatty acid, linoleic acid. The body does not manufacture linoleic acid, so it must be provided by food. Linoleic acid is required for transport and metabolism of fat, and in its absence, the body cannot make fats properly. It is also required for the function and integrity of cell membranes and lowering of serum cholesterol, and prevents and cures skin troubles (dermatitis or eczema) in infants. Fat supplies oils in the skin and hair follicles, which prevent dryness and give the complexion a healthy glow. In cooking, fats add taste to foods and make meals satisfying because fats digest slowly and delay a feeling of hunger. (Problems of high fat consumption are discussed in Chapter 5 on "Natural Diet.")

Common sources of fat are cooking oils (butter, margarine, shortening), cream, nuts, bacon and other fatty meats. Regular meats, whole milk, eggs and chocolate also contain some fat.

Minerals: Minerals are another basic component of nutrition needs. They give strength and rigidity to certain body tissues and are needed for normal metabolism. They must be present in the diet in sufficient amounts for the maintenance of good health. The human body contains relatively small amounts of individual minerals. Collectively, these form 4 to 5 percent of body weight. The ultimate source of minerals for all living things, from plants to humans, is the soil. There are 21 mineral elements now known to be essential in nutrition. The minerals of the body are calcium, phosphorus, sulfur, potassium, chlorine, sodium, magnesium, iron, fluorine, zinc, copper, iodine, chromium, cobalt, silicon, vanadium, tin, selenium, manganese, nickel and molybdenum in order of decreasing amounts in the adult body. As will be discussed next, some of the particularly important minerals are calcium, phosphorus, sulfur, magnesium, sodium, chlorine, potassium, iron, iodine, and fluorine.

Calcium: The body needs calcium throughout life, but especially during periods of growth, pregnancy and lactation. Calcium is the most abundant mineral element in the body and teamed up with phosphorus is responsible for hardness of bones and teeth. About 99 percent of the calcium in the body is found in these two tissues. In the bones, calcium occurs in the form of a salt called hydroxyapatite, which is composed of calcium phosphate and calcium carbonate arranged in a characteristic crystal structure around a framework of softer protein material. It is the hydroxyapatite which provides rigidity and strength to the bones and teeth. The remaining 1 percent of the body's calcium is found in the body fluids and soft tissues. This calcium, present principally in ionic form, has important metabolic functions such as blood clotting, transport function of cell membranes, nerve transmission, regulation of heart beat, and activity of the enzyme ATP (adenosine triphosphate) in the release of energy for muscular contraction. Milk is an abundant source of calcium; but calcium is also found in good amounts in certain darkgreen leafy vegetables such as collards, turnip greens, broccoli, kale, spinach, and mustard greens. Other good sources of calcium are sardines, clams, and oysters.

Phosphorus: Second to calcium in abundance, phosphorus receives little attention by nutritionists because it is a universal cell component available in all foods. About 80 percent of phosphorus is present in association with calcium as insoluble calcium phosphate (apatite) crystals in bones and teeth. One gram of phosphorus is required for every two grams of calcium retained. The other 20 percent is very active metabolically, and has more functions than any other mineral element. Phosphorus is an essential component of nucleic acids, and phospholipids of cell membranes. It plays an important role in phosphorylation of many compounds such as glucose for their utilization in metabolic reactions. The phosphate buffer system helps in regulation of body fluids, including the tubular fluids of the kidney. Phosphorus is supplied by foods that provide calcium and proteins. Milk and milk products are good sources, as are nuts and legumes including cereals and grains. Meat, poultry, fish, and eggs are other excellent sources of phosphorus.

Sulfur: Sulfur occurs principally as a constituent of amino-acids cystine, cysteine, and methionine, which are present in all the proteins. The proteins particularly high in sulfur are keratin of skin and hair (4 to 6 percent sulfur), and insulin (3.2 percent sulfur) which regulates carbohydrate metabolism. Sulfur also occurs in carbohydrates such as heparin, an anticoagulant found in liver. Chondroitin sulfate in bone and cartilage is another place for sulfur. Two vitamins, thiamin and biotin, contain sulfur. The dietary sources for sulfur are protein foods such as meat, fish, poultry, eggs, milk, cheese, legumes, and nuts.

Magnesium: A large amount (about 60 percent) of magnesium is found in bones and teeth. Among other places, 26 percent is found in muscle, and the remainder in soft tissues and body fluids. Along with phosphorus, magnesium plays an important role in the body's use of food for energy. It is essential for protein synthesis, for contractility of muscle, excitability in nerves, and as a cofactor in numerous enzyme systems. Magnesium is found in nuts, whole grain products, dry beans, dry peas, and dark-green vegetables (as an essential constituent of chlorophyll). Other sources are seafood, cocoa and chocolate. High calcium, protein or vitamin D intake as well as alcohol consumption increase magnesium requirements.

Sodium, Chlorine, Potassium: These three elements are discussed together because of their related functions in the body. Sodium, chlorine and potassium are involved in at least four important physiological functions of the body: (1) maintenance of normal water balance and distribution (2) maintenance of normal osmotic equilibrium (3) maintenance of normal acid-base balance (4) maintenance of normal muscular irritability. Sodium constitutes 2 percent, chlorine 3 percent, and potassium 5 percent of the total mineral content of the body. These are distributed throughout all body fluids and tissues. The need for sodium chloride, a common table salt, has been known ever since man has been living on this planet. Deficiency of sodium chloride occurs mainly during hot weather or as a result of heavy work in a hot climate when excessive sweating takes place. Water intoxication can occur if a large quantity of water is taken without added salt. Sodium, chlorine and potassium are all readily absorbed in the intestine and excreted primarily through the urine and sweat. The blood sodium level is controlled in two ways. When blood sodium levels rise, the thirst sensation is stimulated, and when blood sodium levels are low, the excretion of sodium through the urine decreases. It is frequently necessary to restrict sodium intake in order to control the over retention of body water in various pathological states, particularly hypertension (high blood pressure). The exact role of sodium in hypertension is not clear, but it appears that susceptibility to salt-induced hypertension is genetic (for further discussion, see "salt" in later section on "Controversial Chemicals" in this Chapter). In addition to common table salt used in foods, sodium and chlorine are provided in sea foods, meat, milk and eggs. Vegetables and fruits are low in these elements. Potassium is found in fruits, milk, meat, cereals, vegetables, and legumes.

Iron: Sixty to seventy percent of iron in the human body exists as functional iron, most of which is in hemoglobin of erythrocytes; and thirty to forty percent exists as storage iron primarily in the liver, bone marrow and spleen. Iron combines with protein to make hemoglobin, the red substance of blood that carries oxygen from the lungs to body cells and removes carbon dioxide from the cells. Iron also plays an important role in the process of cellular respiration and helps the cells obtain energy from food. The foods that provide iron include liver, oysters, shellfish, kidney, heart, dry beans, dry peas, dark-green vegetables, dried fruit, egg yolk and smaller amounts in whole-grain and enriched bread and cereals. Milk and milk products are practically devoid of iron.

Fluorine: The most familiar beneficial effect of fluorine is the protection against dental cavities. The skeleton of an average person contains 2.6 grams of fluorine. Studies have demonstrated that the hydroxyapatite crystals in bones are larger and more nearly perfect when the fluoride content of the diet is adequate. Bone containing fluoride is more stable and more resistant to degeneration. Fluorine usually occurs in drinking water naturally or is added to it, and use of such water makes teeth more resistant to decay. While pills, drugs and fluoridated tooth paste are of some use, none attain the efficiency, effectiveness and the economy of water fluoridation.

Table 3.3 Mineral elements requirements and likelihood of deficiency.

Mineral	Adult daily requirement	Likelihood of deficiency
Macronutrients required 100 mg or more per day		
Calcium	800 mg	Since bone serves as homeostatic mechanism to maintain calcium level in blood, dietary deficiency can occur only after a long term depletion of calcium in diet.
Phosphorus	800 mg	Dietary deficiency not likely to occur if protein and calcium intake is adequate.
Sulfur	Need satisfied by sulfur-containing amino acids	Adequacy related to protein intake because dietary intake is chiefly from sulfur-containing amino acids of a protein.
Magnesium	350 mg	Dietary inadequacy unlikely, but conditioned deficiency due to alcoholism, malabsorption, loss of body fluids can occur.
Sodium	2,500 mg	Dietary inadequacy unlikely.
Chlorine	2,000 mg	Dietary inadequacy unlikely.
Potassium	2,500 mg	Dietary inadequacy unlikely.
Micronutrients required a few milligrams per day		
Iron	10 mg	Iron-deficiency anemia likely in reproductive women, infants and preschool children.
Iodine	14 mg	Iodized salts helpful in areas of low iodine foods.
Fluorine	not established	Fluoridation of water helpful in areas of low fluorine water.
Zinc	15 mg	Dietary inadequacy uncommon.
Copper	No recommended amount but 2 mg adequate	No deficiencies known.
Maganese Molybdenum Cobalt, selenium, Chromium	Not established	Deficiencies unlikely.

Iodine: About 60 percent of iodine is in the thyroid glands and the rest is diffused throughout all tissues. The only known function of iodine is as an integral part of thyroid hormones, which themselves carry out a variety of functions. These hormones regulate growth, energy transformation through an effect on oxygen consumption and heat production, reproduction, neuromuscular function, skin and hair growth, and cellular metabolism. The reliable sources of iodine are iodized salts and seafoods.

In addition to iron, fluorine and iodine, the rest of the micronutrients such as zinc, copper, chromium, cobalt, silicon, vanadium, tin, selenium, manganese, nickel, and molybdenum form a part of many enzymes and are required in very small amounts. In the absence of these micronutrients, enzymes, which are required for important metabolic processes such as digestion, will not function properly. These metals function in enzymes by direct participation in catalysis, combination with substrate to form a complex upon which the enzyme acts, formation of a metalloenzyme which binds substrate, combination of metal with a reaction product, and maintenance of quaternary structure. These important minerals not described individually are usually provided in satisfactory amounts by a well chosen variety of foods.

The recommended dietary allowances of various mineral elements for healthy adults, and comments on likelihood of deficiency are listed in Table 3.3.

Vitamins: Vitamins, which are present in small quantities in foods in their natural state, are essential for normal metabolism and for the development and maintenance of tissue structure and function. With a few exceptions the body cannot synthesize vitamins; they must be supplied in the diet or in addition to the diet. Certain vitamins such as vitamin K, thiamin, folacin and B_{12} may be formed by microorganisms in the intestinal tract, and it is known that vitamin A, choline and niacine can be formed if their precursors are supplied. Vitamin D can be synthesized in the skin upon exposure to sunlight. In the case of supplement vitamin use, synthetic vitamins are as good as natural vitamins. Although natural vitamins cost twice as much as synthetic, there is no evidence for the superiority of natural vitamins over synthetic ones. A dozen or more major vitamins have been identified. These are divided into two groups on the basis of solubility; the fat-soluble vitamins such as vitamins A, D, E, and K, and water-soluble vitamins such as B-complex and C. The excessive intake of fat-soluble vitamins will result in increased storage of vitamins, which has little or no beneficial effect, but rather, taken to extreme, may cause toxicity (see Chapter 5 on "Natural Diet"). Water-soluble vitamins, however, are not stored, but excessive intake, regularly, may create dependency. Healthy persons who eat well-balanced meals including sufficient vegetables and fruits, rarely require vitamins as medication. However, over-cooking can result in loss of vitamins from the food. A good rule to follow is to avoid long cooking at high temperature in the presence of air or under alkaline conditions, and to use as little water as is feasible. The potency of vitamins is also related to their length of shelf storage time.

Vitamin A (Retinol): Vitamin A has been named retinol because it serves a specific function in the retina of the eye. Vitamin A is a constituent of the visual purple (rhodopsin) of the retina, and is necessary for normal dim light vision. Deficiency of vitamin A results in night blindness. An injection of vitamin A corrects this condition within a matter of minutes. Vision defects such as color blindness are genetic and cannot be cured by vitamin A. This vitamin is also necessary for growth and development of skeletal and soft tissues. Vitamin A helps normal bone development and tooth formation in early life. Animal studies have shown that vitamin A is required to assure normal reproduction and lactation. It also helps keep the skin and inner linings of the body healthy and resistant to infection. Vitamin A is found in liver, kidney, eggs, butter, margarine, whole milk, and in vegetables and fruits which are dark-green and deep-yellow. The dark-green and deep-yellow vegetables and fruits contain a substance carotene that the body can change into vitamin A. Cod and halibut fish oils are usually sources for therapeutic doses of vitamin A.

Vitamin D (Calciferol):   Vitamin D is important in building strong bones and teeth because it enables the body to use the calcium and phosphorus supplied by food. In infants and children, deficiency of vitamin D results in malformation of bones due to low deposition of calcium phosphate (hydroxyapatite), the disease which is called rickets. In the adult, low vitamin D cause decalcification of the bone shafts which makes bones vulnerable to fracture. However, bending of bones in adults does not occur, because bones are already formed. The important source of vitamin D is milk with added vitamin D. Other sources are sardines, salmon, herring, tuna, egg yolk, butter, and liver. Vitamin D is also produced by action of direct sunlight on the skin.

Vitamin E (Tocopherol):   Vitamin E is an antioxidant and appears to protect the membranes from deterioration caused by peroxidation of membrane lipid. The ability of vitamin E to protect the membrane lipid has been related to delaying the aging process (see Chapter 6 on "Aging"). Lack of vitamin E has been suggested to produce sterility in both sexes, loss of hair, miscarriage, muscle weakness, and muscular dystrophy. The richest source of vitamin E is wheat germ oil. The other sources are cereal germs, green vegetables (such as lettuce, parsley, spinach, turnip leaf), egg yolk, milk fat, butter, liver meats, nuts, and vegetable oils.

Vitamin K (Menadione):   Vitamin K is essential for the synthesis of several proteins involved in the clotting of blood. Frequently, it is given to patients before surgery to prevent abnormal bleeding. Vitamin K is found in green leafy vegetables, especially cabbage, spinach, kale and lettuce. It is also found in cauliflower, tomatoes, wheat bran, soybeans, oil, cheese, egg yolk and liver. Vitamin K has been shown to be formed by bacterial action found in the lower intestinal tract, so that an important supply of this vitamin may be available even if it is not supplied in the diet.

Vitamin B-complex: Originally, vitamin B was recognized as the preventive factor in the disease beriberi. To date more than a dozen separate B vitamins have been identified and found to play important roles in nutrition. The members of the B-complex group are commonly referred to by their chemical names. Thiamin is B_1, riboflavin is B_2, pyridoxine is B_6, and we also have niacin (nicotinic acid), pantothenic acid, folacin, biotin, inositol and choline. The B group, in general, plays an essential role in the metabolic processes of all living cells by serving as cofactors in the various enzyme systems involved in the oxidation of food and production of energy. In other words, the B group vitamins provide components vital to the transformation of food into energy by the cells of the body. Other functions include healthy skin, normal appetite, good digestion and proper functioning of nerves. In addition to organ meats such as liver, these vitamins are found in milk, whole grain and cereals. The rich source for riboflavin is milk, for thiamin lean pork, and for niacin protein rich in essential amino acid tryptophan. The tryptophan can be changed into niacin by the body. Other B vitamins such as B_6 and B_{12} and folacin help prevent anemia. These are found in organ meats, leafy green vegetables, whole grain cereals, dry beans, and potatoes.

Vitamin C (Ascorbic Acid): Though vitamin C is stored in small amounts in the liver, intestinal walls and adrenal cortex, it must be replenished daily. Vitamin C is the antiscorbutic vitamin, the preventive of and cure for scurvy, the dreaded disease of early explorers and voyagers. It requires about 3 months for scurvy to develop in a person on a vitamin C deficient diet. Scurvy is characterized by general debility, pallor, poor appetite, sensitivity to touch, pains in the limbs and joints, especially the knee joints, sensitive and swollen gums, with bleeding and loosening of the teeth. Vitamin C or ascorbic acid is familiar to many of us as a vitamin thought to prevent common cold in some mysterious way. As an antioxidant, it is associated with slowing down the aging process (see Chapter 6 on "Aging"). It helps form and maintain cementing material that holds body cells together and strengthens the walls of blood vessels. It also assists in normal tooth and bone formation and aids in healing wounds. Citrus fruits such as oranges, grapefruit, lemons and fresh strawberries are rich sources of ascorbic acid. Other sources are tomatoes, broccoli, brussels sprouts, cabbage, cantaloupe, cauliflower, green peppers, dark-green leafy vegeatbles, and watermelon.

Table 3.4 summarizes the daily recommended allowances of various vitamins for adults, and information on pharmaceutical sources and stability of vitamins to cooking and other storage or environmental conditions.

Water: Water is not really a food in the fuel or calorie-producing sense but it ranks next to air (oxygen) in importance as a fundamental requirement of life. About 55 to 65 percent of the body weight is made up of water. The distribution of body water is not fixed and can vary under different conditions, but the total amount in the body remains relatively constant. Water is the solvent in which all of the metabolic changes take place; it functions in digestion, absorption, circulation and excretion. Water plays a role in the maintenance of body temperature. The evaporation of perspiration keeps the body cool. Water acts as a transporting medium for nutrients and all body substances. Metabolic waste products

Table 3.4 Vitamins requirements, and their stability to cooking and other environmental conditions.

Vitamin	Daily adult requirements	Pharmaceutical sources	Stability
Fat-soluble vitamins			
A (Retinol)	5,000 I.U. (2 eggs)	Fish liver oil.	Stable to light, heat and normal cooking.
D (Calciferol)	400 I.U.	Fish liver oil, concentrates.	Stable to heat and oxidation.
E (Tocopherol)	15 I.U.	Wheat germ oil, synthetic.	Stable to heat and acids.
K (Menadione)	Not established dose of 1–2 mg adequate.	Synthetic	Stable to heat, oxygen and moisture.
Water-soluble vitamins			
B_1 (Thiamin)	1.0–1.4 mg	Yeast, wheat germ, synthetic.	Unstable to heat, alkali or oxygen.
B_2 (Riboflavin)	1.4–1.8 mg	Yeast, liver concentrates, synthetic.	Stable to heat, oxygen and acid.
Niacin (Nicotinic acid)	13–18 mg	Yeast, liver concentrate, synthetic.	Stable to heat, light, oxidation, acid and alkali.
B_6 (Pyridoxine)	2.0 mg	Yeast, wheat germ, liver concentrates.	Stable to heat, light and oxidation.
Pantothenic acid	10.0 mg	Yeast, wheat germ, liver concentrates.	Unstable to acid, alkali, heat and certain salts.
H (Biotin)	Unknown but 0.1 to 0.3 mg adequate	Yeast, liver concentrates.	Stable.
Folacin (Folic acid)	0.4 mg	Yeast concentrates.	Stable to sunlight.
B_{12} (Cyano-cobalamin)	3 microgram (0.003 mg)	Concentrates, synthetic.	Slowly destroyed by acid, alkali, light and oxidation.
C (Ascorbic acid)	45 mg (1 orange)	Synthetic	Unstable to heat, alkali, and oxidation. Destroyed by storage.

generated in the cells of the body are transported in the water solution via the blood to the kidneys where the wastes are excreted in urine. Water serves as a building material for growth and repair of the body. It is a part of all body tissues and fluids. Water in the intestinal tract aids elimination. Water is constantly being eliminated in the form of urine, perspiration and expired breath and it must therefore be replaced regularly to maintain the balance. Thirst tells us more need for water and excretion regulates excessive intake of water. Average adult consumes 1.5 to 2.0 liters of fluids daily. In addition to water itself, beverages, fruits, vegetables and meats, all supply water to various extents. Water is also formed when the body uses food for energy during oxidation process. The oxidation of 100 gram of fat, carbohydrate or protein yields 107, 55 and 41 gram of water, respectively.

Some Controversial Chemicals

Cholesterol, salt, sugar, alcohol, caffeine and nicotine are the subjects of the most intense and persistent controversy in human health today. Vast amounts of scientific and statistical data indicate that these substances are related to a high risk of certain serious problems. Although more studies are still needed to collect more direct proof for some of the claims, concern seems to be serious enough so that education regarding their physical effects and potential danger is important for those who are concerned about their health. People need to learn how to use them, if at all, sensibly and in moderation.

Cholesterol: Cholesterol, which is often associated with fats, is not itself a fat. It is a member of the large group of compounds called sterols. It is more like a wax and does not dissolve easily in water or blood plasma, a property similar to a fat. Cholesterol is found not only as a free sterol but also in combination with fatty acids, as esters. It is found only in animal tissue and is an essential component of the structural membranes of all cells and is a major component of brain and nerve cells. Cholesterol helps make bile acids for digestion and steroid hormones such as progesterone (one of the sex hormones involved in development of secondary sex characteristics). Cholesterol in the skin along with other lipids makes the skin resistant to the action of many chemical agents.

Although cholesterol is an essential body chemical, it arouses controversy because excessive cholesterol is associated with several conditions including atherosclerosis, hypertension and diabetes. When too much cholesterol gets into the blood, it takes the form of plaques, which settle into artery walls, hardening and narrowing them. As the plaques get larger and larger, the opening through which the blood must flow gets narrower and narrower. Eventually circulation through an artery can be completely blocked. If the artery happens to be one that nourishes the heart, the result is a heart attack, and it is frequently fatal. A similar blockage in an artery feeding the brain can result in a stroke. Clogged arteries in the legs can result in painful muscle spasms resulting from even slight exercise because with reduced circulation, the muscles cannot get enough oxygen (which is carried in the blood).

The body cholesterol level is influenced by *lipoproteins* which are important to its transport. Since cholesterol-like fat is not soluble in the blood, it must be carried in the blood by the lipoproteins that are formed in the liver. Three main types of lipoproteins control the cholesterol transport. High-density lipoproteins (HDL) prevent atherosclerosis by removing cholesterol from artery walls and returning it to the liver for excretion. Two other types of cholesterol carriers, the low-density lipoproteins (LDL) and the very-low-density lipoproteins (VLDL), have the opposite effect. They keep the cholesterol in circulation, passing through the arteries, and this is how the arteries become clogged with cholesterol deposits.

Although cholesterol is not a fat, the popular association of it with fat is due to the fact that dietary fat intake has a direct effect on the serum cholesterol level of an individual. In fact the amount of cholesterol circulating in blood is influenced more by the amount and kind of fats one consumes than by the dietary cholesterol intake. The total concentration of cholesterol in the blood plasma is highly variable, averaging about 200 mg per 100 ml in the adult. Although many medical communities use cholesterol 'norms' up to 300, a level of 100 to 200 is considered more appropriate for good health.

Reduced intake of fats, particularly the saturated ones, (see section on "Fats" in this Chapter), along with reduced intake of dietary cholesterol is the most effective way to avoid the cholesterol-associated risk of heart problems. Cholesterol occurs in greatest amounts in egg yolk and organ meats such as liver, kidney, and brain. In addition, all animal fats which are generally saturated contain cholesterol, but no cholesterol is naturally present in any of the vegetable foods. For this reason, the natural diet described in Chapter 5 places special emphasis on the importance of vegetable foods to avoid dangers of excessive fats and cholesterol intake.

Salt: The need for common table salt, sodium chloride, is mentioned earlier in the mineral section under sodium, chlorine, and potassium. It primarily helps to maintain water balance, osmotic equilibrium, acid-base balance, and muscular irritability. It is needed to avoid water intoxication when the intake of large quantities of water is made necessary by hot weather or heavy work in a hot climate. It requires special attention as a controversial chemical, because for four decades, we have known that dietary salt contributes to hypertension. The exact role of salt in hypertension is not clear, but it could lead to over-retention of body water. With additional water weight, the heart has to work harder and also the salt-caused edema (swelling) creates extra pressure against the vessel walls.

Although a condition of hypertension is suggested to be genetic, at least in some cases, people with high salt intake, generally, demonstrate a higher frequency of hypertension. The northern Japanese, for example, eat three times as much salt as Americans do and 40 percent of them have hypertension as compared to 20 percent of Americans. Low-salt eaters such as Eskimos, have low rates of hypertension. Therefore, low salt intake, is an advisable step, particularly for those with family history of hypertension.

The average salt intake for Americans is 6 to 18 grams daily, much of which is added to foods. Present evidence indicates that 0.6 to 3.5 gram is an adequate daily intake. This can be supplied by the natural salt present in varying amounts in almost all foods. Excessive salt intake in American infants is a more severe problem than in adults because infants consume a higher proportion of commercially prepared and processed foods, as determined by the Committee of Nutrition of the American Academy of Pediatrics.

Lowering fats and raising carbohydrates in the diet as suggested in Chapter 5 on "Natural Diet," can reduce hypertension—even if 9 to 10 grams of salt is consumed everyday. A natural diet will also reduce the dangers of excess salt intake supplied, particularly, by commercially prepared and processed foods.

Sugar: Sugar is one of the carbohydrates—the major sources of energy for humans. Although carbohydrates from starch-rich natural foods are imperative to maintain a good health (as you will realize later in Chapter 5 on "Natural Diet"), the refined carbohydrates such as sugar are actually a threat to good health.

While the most popular sweetener is common table sugar, several other sugars are consumed under various names. Table sugar, sucrose, is a disaccharide composed of fructose and glucose. Other disaccharide sugars are lactose (milk sugar) and maltose (malt sugar), which are composed of glucose-galactose and glucose-glucose, respectively. The disaccharides may be broken down by the body into monosaccharides using enzymes sucrase, lactase, and maltase. The other sugars which occur as monosaccharides are glucose (blood sugar), fructose (fruit sugar) and galactose (produced from milk sugar). In addition to the pure monosaccharides and disaccharides, there are less purified sugars such as honey, molasses, brown sugar and corn or maple syrup.

Any of the concentrated sugars including sucrose (table sugar), honey, and various syrups have deleterious effects in excessive quantity. The only beneficial effect that of providing concentrated calories for energy, may be deleterious, particularly to an obese person. Sugar consumption, which in America contributes an average of 24 percent of total caloric intake, is an important factor in overweight problem. Because sugar is highly refined, it lacks vitamins, minerals, and fiber, and also makes you eat more calories than your body uses up. For example, three pounds of sugar beets, which in addition to sugar cane are the common sources of table sugar, contribute the same amount of calories as 1/3 pound of pure sugar (average one day consumption) extracted from them. In addition, sugar beets provide excellent nutrition and fiber as well as satisfy your appetite. Among other negative effects of sugar, the connection between sweets and dental cavities is a commonly known health hazard of sugar. Sugar also seems to raise the level of blood fats and cholesterol both of which promote atherosclerosis by clogging arteries. Sugar has also been blamed for hypoglycemia or low blood sugar. For instance, when food is eaten, the blood sugar level rises, and in response to this rise in blood sugar, the body produces a hormone, insulin. The insulin then clears the blood of excess sugar by delivering it to body cells where it is used for energy or converted to fat for storage. In certain people, the body overreacts to an excessive rise of sugar and produces far too much insulin to clear it, which results in a lower sugar level in the blood. The low blood sugar causes feelings of lightheadedness, fatigue, weakness and so forth. The close relationship between sugar and insulin levels is well known in diabetes, when the pancreas fail to produce adequate amounts of insulin in response to a rise in blood sugar.

In any case, the less the sugar, the better it is. Almost any amount of sugar is too much. The simple tip to reduce sugar consumption is to stick with natural foods (as emphasized later in Chapter 5) because three-fourth of the sugar we eat come in processed foods. Serving fresh fruits for desserts and elimination of soft drinks from the diet can significantly reduce sugar intake. The use of saccharin or other artificial sweeteners to replace sugar is not a wise step in view of reports giving rise to the suspicion that bladder cancer may be caused by saccharin.

Alcohol: Alchohol means different things to different people—it may be valued as a food, a medicine, a drug, or a ceremonial drink. Although alcohol in itself is a food in the sense that its caloric content produces energy in the body, it contains practically no essential nutrients. Beer or wine are exceptions in that they include unfermented carbohydrates-sugars and starches in addition to alcohol. Chemically, the alcohol used for drinks is ethyl alcohol. It is produced by the natural process of fermentation of certain foods such as fruits, grains or their juices. When these foods are left in a warm place for a sufficient amount of time, airborne yeast organisms begin to change the sugars and starches into alcohol. Since alcohol has a lower boiling point than water, it can be separated from the fermented foods by a process of distillation. Soon after the process of distillation was discovered, it was applied to wine to make brandy and to the various beers based on rye, corn, and barley to make whiskies.

Alcohol has several effects upon the human body, some of which may be quite familiar to many of us. In general, it is known that in moderate quantities, alcohol causes the following reactions: the heartbeat quickens slightly, appetite increases, and gastric juices are stimulated. In other words, a drink makes people "feel good."

Alcohol, however, has many negative effects on our health. Habitual drinking of, for example, straight whiskey, can irritate the membranes that line the mouth and the throat. As for the effect on the stomach, alcohol does not cause ulcers, but it does aggravate them. Alcohol is damaging to the liver, and chronic users have an increased risk of liver disease (cirrhosis). Unfortunately, heavy drinkers, consuming large amounts of empty calories, pay little attention to their nutrition and often suffer from malnutrition. The brain damage observed in chronic alcoholics has been attributed to the absence from the diet of essential proteins and vitamins rather than alcohol itself. However, the moderate use of alcoholic beverages has no proven permanent effect on brain or nerve tissue. Heavy drinkers also have lower immunity to infection, increased susceptibility to irritation of urinary tract and the prostate, and even a shorter life span than others. The most common effects of chronic alcoholism are disorders of the central nervous system. There may be tremors of the hands, deterioration of eye function, and suffering of bladder control. Changes in behavior result from a decrease in inhibition control: excessive cheerfulness quickly turns into weeping; moods of self-hatred alternate with moods of hostility to others. The attention span grows shorter, and there are increasing lapses of memory.

None of the problems of heavy drinkers, however, apply to a moderate drinker. In fact the statistics for moderate drinkers have shown that they live longer than those who don't drink at all. However, in this connection it has been pointed out that those who drink sensibly are likely to have equally good judgment in other health matters. Alcohol, by depressing inhibition centers of the brain, is claimed to stimulate sexual pleasure, but many unwanted pregnancies, particularly among young pepople, are also associated with drinking because of impairment of judgment. Sometimes doctors suggest it as a medicine to induce sleep and to stimulate appetite. The combination of alcoholic beverages with drugs such as sedatives and sleep-producing (barbiturates) drugs, and tranquilizers (calm without producing sleep) should be carefully avoided. Such combinations of chemicals in the system can be fatal.

We can safely conclude from the above discussion that the drinking of excessive alcohol is certainly bad and drinking moderate amounts or no alcohol is the path to follow. The excessive use of alcohol, in fact, is a serious problem and the loss of control over drinking behavior is considered a disease, which is familiar to us by the name "alcoholism." Alcohol doesn't cause alcoholism. Nor is it an inherited illness. The causes of alcoholism include physiological, psychological, and sociological factors such as marital, financial, and job problems. The common danger signals of a problem drinker include: (1) Increasing use of alcohol with repeated occasions of unintended intoxication; (2) Sneaking drinks or gulping them rapidly in quick succession; (3) Irritation, hostility, and lying when the subject of excessive drinking is mentioned (In other words, the alcoholic, generally, does not admit that he is an alcoholic); (4) Persistent drinking in spite of such symptoms as loss of appetite, headaches, sleeplessness, and stomach trouble. If any of your friends or relatives show some of the above symptoms or in your judgment is an alcoholic, the best help you can provide is to convince the person to seek help through a private arrangement or through an agency such as Alcoholics Anonymous.

Caffeine: Caffeine, which is naturally present in coffee and tea and is used in many carbonated beverages and medications, stimulates the central nervous system to overcome fatigue and drowsiness. It also affects a part of the nervous system that controls respiration so that more oxygen is pumped through the lungs. Because of the action of caffeine in stimulating an increased intake of oxygen, it sometimes is used to combat the effects of such nervous system depressants as alcohol. Caffeine can produce various other effects such as increases in metabolic rate, reaction of stomach acids, and urine production.

Too much caffeine has been known to increase pulse rate and even cause irregular heartbeats, ulcers, insomnia, and severe anxiety. The withdrawl of caffeine may sometimes be more effective to control severe cases of anxiety than the use of tranquilizers. Caffeine has also been suspected of contributing to birth defects. Although caffeine drinks are not addictive, withdrawal from an accustomed cup of coffee may give a headache or cause depression for a short time. Tea is generally considered safer than coffee mainly due to its lower caffeine content (Table 3.5). The tannins in tea are a source of concern, because these may cause liver damage. However, the use of tea bags in boiled water reduces the amount of tannins oozing out, and addition of milk also helps to bind the trouble-making tannins. Some of the Indian and Chinese teas contain little or no tannin which sometimes can be judged by the astringent effect on the tongue.

Table 3.5 The caffeine content of various drinks and products.

Product	Serving size	Caffeine (mg)
Coffee		
Brewed drip	6 ounces	175
Brewed percolated	6 ounces	132
Instant regular	6 ounces	64
Decaffeinated	6 ounces	2
Tea		
One-minute brew	6 ounces	11–40
Three-minute brew	6 ounces	24–55
Five-minute brew	6 ounces	24–60
Canned ice tea	12 ounces	22–36
Soft drinks		
Mountain Dew	12 ounces	52
Mellow yellow	12 ounces	51
Tab	12 ounces	44
Sunkist orange	12 ounces	42
Shasta Cola	12 ounces	42
Dr. Pepper	12 ounces	37
Pepsi	12 ounces	37
RC Cola	12 ounces	36
Coca Cola	12 ounces	34
Mr. Pibb	12 ounces	33
7 Up	12 ounces	0
Sprite	12 ounces	0
Fanta	12 ounces	0
Cocoa and Chocolate		
Cocoa beverage	6 ounces	10
Baking chocolate	1 ounce	35
Milk chocolate	1 ounce	6
Nonprescription drugs		
Stimulants		
Caffedrine capsules	standard dose	200
NoDoz Tablets	standard dose	200
Vivarin Tablets	standard dose	200
Pain relievers		
Excedrin	standard dose	130
Anacin	standard dose	64
Midol	standard dose	65
Aspirin	standard dose	0
Diuretics		
Aqua-Ban	standard dose	200
Permathene H_2 Off	standard dose	200
Pre-Mens Forte	standard dose	100
Cold remedies		
Coryban-D	standard dose	30
Dristan	standard dose	32

Table 3.5 Continued.

Product	Serving size	Caffeine (mg)
Triaminicin	standard dose	30
Weight-control aids		
Dexatrim	daily dose	200
Dietac	daily dose	200
Prolamine	daily dose	280

SOURCE: Consumer Reports, 1981.

After learning about the health effects of caffeine, you may have been prompted to cut back on its consumption. Table 3.5 lists the caffeine content of various common drinks and other caffeine sources, which may be helpful in avoiding high caffeine products. Although coffee is the largest source of caffeine, yet soft drinks are not much less of a culprit, ranking second. The soft drinks are a number one beverage in the United States and the average consumption in 1980 was about 34 gallons per person in one year. Tea ranks third as a source of caffeine. The non-prescription drugs such as pain relievers and weight control pills contain large doses of caffeine, even though no scientific evidence supports the role of caffeine in killing pain or reducing weight. Now one way to cut back on caffeine, of course, is to avoid sources of caffeine. The use of instant coffee rather than brewed can reduce the caffeine consumption to about half. Similarly reducing the brewing time for tea can cut down not only the caffeine content but also the tannins. By avoiding soft drinks, you can eliminate caffeine and additives, both of which are hazardous to the health.

Ordinarily, drinking a few cups of coffee or tea (preferably with a little milk) or a caffeine beverage should not be made a main concern. But if you find that you need a caffeine beverage to keep going, you need a rest and should follow the pages of this book very carefully to develop vigor and vitality.

Nicotine (smoking): Nicotine, which is one of many substances present in tobacco, affects the human physiology by stimulating the adrenal glands to increase the flow of adrenaline. The release of adrenaline produces temporary relief from fatigue by increasing the flow of sugar in the blood. Stimulation of adrenal glands also cause blood vessels to constrict and skin temperature to drop.

The well established dangerous effects of tobacco smoking such as lung cancer, heart disease, and emphysema-bronchitis are familiar to many of us. Another less publicized effect of smoking is the accumulation of carbon monoxide in the blood, which is a problem in addition to the devastating effect of nicotine and tar. When carbon monoxide binds to the red blood cell hemoglobin, they form a stable structure, carboxyhemoglobin, which can tie up the red blood cells' oxygen-carrying capacity for up to twelve hours. The shortness of breath among smokers, particularly during exercise is due to this carbon monoxide effect. The oxygen starvation effect on arteries is what appears to be the reason that smokers have a much higher risk of heart disease, stroke, hypertension, angina, and all the other athero-sclerosis-related diseases. Smoking has also been suggested to accelerate some of the symptoms such as osteoporosis generally associated with old age.

The only solution to reduce the dangers of smoke-related-problems is to stop smoking. Some experts believe that after about a decade of nonsmoking, a former smoker's risk equals that of a lifelong nonsmoker in many areas of risk. Although there are various articles and books suggesting tips on how to give up smoking, the crucial first step is the personal motivation, which may be gained through an awareness of self-health as emphasized throughout this book.

Safty Tips Against Controversial Chemicals: The best safety against the potential health hazards of chemicals, cholesterol, salt, sugar, caffeine, alcohol, and nico-tine, of course, is to stop or reduce their use. The consumption of the first four of these can be easily reduced by sensible control over use of their sources. The alcohol and smoking (nicotine), however, need particular consideration.

Before considering the use of nutrients to provide protection against undesirable *alcohol* effects, let us consider the metabolic aspect of alcohol. The enzyme called alcohol dehydrogenase converts alcohol to acetaldehyde, a chemical which can damage the body in several ways. However, our bodies have another enzyme called dehydrogenase which oxidizes the toxic acetaldehyde into essentially harm-less acetate (a form of common vinegar). The problem of acetaldehyde danger arises only when excessive amount of alcohol is consumed. Researchers have observed that a combination of certain nutrients can provide protection against acetaldehyde. These nutrients include vitamins C and B_1 and the amino-acid cysteine. You may have heard the old remedy for a hangover: a raw egg stirred into a large glass of orange juice. The egg contains about 250 milligrams (0.25 gram) of cysteine, and the large glass of orange juice about 250 milligrams of vitamin C. The doses as high as 1 gram each of cysteine and vitamin B_1 and 5 grams of vitamin C have been suggested for heavy drinkers.

If you are a *smoker*, you know, of course, that nothing can be safer than quit-ting smoking. However, you can reduce the risks of smoking by using the nutrient supplements. We know that nicotine causes blood vessels to constrict, thus in-creasing blood pressure. It also causes an increase in blood fats, such as choles-terol. But these effects can be largely countered with niacin (also called nicotinic acid or vitamin B_3); niacin causes dilation of blood vessels and reduction in blood fats. The doses suggested are 0.1 gram to 1 gram of niacin taken 3 times a day on a full stomach. Large doses can many times be annoying due to the acidic nature of this vitamin and its dilation effect on blood vessels. Since cigarette smoke contains heavy metals and carbon monoxide and nitrogen oxide; the dan-gerous effects of these heavy metals and gases can be reduced by using sensible amounts of vitamins A, E and C and minerals selenium (80 microgram) and zinc (see Tables 3.3 and 3.4 for amount guidelines).

Chapter 4

Weight Control and Calories

To maintain a desirable weight is good, not only in terms of good looks, but more important, in terms of good health. Probably the most important dietary problem talked about and written about today is obesity. The problem is a new one: never before has man had so wide a choice—or so regular a supply—of good food; neither did he have such a common use of vehicles that even a natural exercise such as walking would need special efforts. The consequences surround us in a mass of ailments, from obesity to varicose veins and heart disease. In the United States alone more than 10 billion dollars are spent annually on weight reduction efforts of one kind or another.

Overweight or Obesity

Overweight or obesity is a condition of the body in which there is an excessive deposit of fat. Tables 4.1 and 4.2 list the desirable weight for men and women of

Table 4.1 Desirable weights for men of ages 25 and over.

Height		Weight (in indoor clothing)					
		Small Frame		Medium Frame		Large Frame	
(in)	(cm)	(lb)	(kg)	(lb)	(kg)	(lb)	(kg)
61	155	112–120	51–54	118–120	54–59	126–141	57–64
62	158	115–123	52–55	121–123	55–60	129–144	59–65
63	160	118–126	54–57	124–136	56–62	132–148	60–67
64	163	121–129	55–59	127–139	58–63	135–152	61–69
65	165	124–133	56–60	130–143	59–65	138–156	63–71
66	168	128–137	58–62	134–147	61–67	142–161	64–73
67	170	132–141	60–64	138–152	63–69	147–166	67–75
68	173	136–145	62–66	142–156	64–71	151–170	69–77
69	175	140–150	64–68	146–160	66–73	155–174	70–79
70	178	144–154	65–70	150–165	68–75	159–179	72–81
71	180	148–158	67–72	154–170	70–77	164–184	74–84
72	183	152–162	69–74	158–175	72–79	168–189	76–86
73	185	156–167	71–76	162–180	74–82	173–194	79–88
74	188	160–171	73–78	167–185	76–84	178–199	81–90
75	191	164–175	74–79	172–190	78–86	182–204	83–93

SOURCE: Based on "Supplement to How to Control Your Weight," Metropolitan Life Booklet, New York, 1963.

Table 4.2 Desirable weights for women of ages 25 and over.*

| Height | | Weight (in indoor clothing) | | | | | |
| | | Small Frame | | Medium Frame | | Large Frame | |
(in)	(cm)	(lb)	(kg)	(lb)	(kg)	(lb)	(kg)
56	142	92– 98	42–45	96–107	44–49	104–119	47–54
57	145	94–101	43–46	98–110	45–50	106–122	48–55
58	147	96–104	44–47	101–113	46–51	109–125	49–57
59	150	99–107	45–49	104–116	47–53	112–128	51–58
60	152	102–110	46–50	107–119	49–54	115–131	52–59
61	155	105–113	47–51	110–122	50–55	118–134	54–61
62	158	108–116	49–53	113–126	51–57	121–138	55–63
63	160	111–119	50–54	116–130	53–59	125–142	58–64
64	163	114–123	52–56	120–135	54–61	129–146	59–66
65	165	118–127	54–58	124–139	56–63	133–150	60–68
66	168	122–131	55–59	128–143	58–65	137–154	62–70
67	170	126–135	57–61	132–147	60–68	141–158	64–72
68	173	130–140	59–64	136–151	62–69	145–163	66–74
69	175	134–144	61–65	140–155	64–70	149–168	68–76
70	178	138–148	63–67	144–159	65–72	153–173	69–79

*For girls between 18 and 25, subtract 1 pound for each year under 25
SOURCE: Based on "Supplement to How to Control Your Weight," Metropolitan
Life Booklet, New York, 1963.

Table 4.3 Height and weight for boys age 2 to 18 years.

| Age (years) | Height | | | | | | Weight | | | | | |
| | Small | | Medium | | Large | | Small | | Medium | | Large | |
	(in)	(cm)	(in)	(cm)	(in)	(cm)	(lb)	(kg)	(lb)	(kg)	(lb)	(kg)
2	32	82	34	86	37	93	24	11	29	13	35	16
3	35	89	37	95	40	102	26	12	33	15	40	18
4	38	96	41	103	43	110	31	14	37	17	44	20
5	40	102	43	110	46	117	33	15	42	19	51	23
6	43	108	46	116	49	124	37	17	46	21	60	27
7	45	113	48	122	51	130	42	19	51	23	66	30
8	47	118	50	127	54	136	44	20	55	25	77	35
9	48	123	52	132	56	142	49	22	62	28	88	40
10	50	128	54	137	58	148	53	24	71	32	99	45
11	52	132	56	143	61	155	60	27	77	35	115	52
12	54	137	59	149	64	162	66	30	88	40	128	58
13	56	143	61	156	67	169	75	34	99	45	143	65
14	58	148	64	163	69	176	84	38	112	51	159	72
15	61	155	67	169	72	182	95	43	126	57	174	79
16	63	161	68	174	73	185	106	48	137	62	190	86
17	65	165	69	176	74	187	115	52	148	67	203	92
18	65	166	70	177	74	188	119	54	152	69	212	96

SOURCE: Based on data from National Center for Health Statistics: NCHS Growth
Charts, Health Resources Administration, Rockville, Maryland, 1976.

Table 4.4 Height and weight for girls age 2 to 18 years.

Age (years)	Height						Weight					
	Small		Medium		Large		Small		Medium		Large	
	(in)	(cm)	(in)	(cm)	(in)	(cm)	(lb)	(kg)	(lb)	(kg)	(lb)	(kg)
2	32	81	34	86	37	93	22	10	26	12	31	14
3	35	88	37	94	40	101	26	12	31	14	37	17
4	37	95	40	102	43	108	29	13	35	16	44	20
5	40	101	43	108	46	116	33	15	40	18	51	23
6	42	107	45	115	48	123	35	16	44	20	57	26
7	44	112	48	121	51	129	40	18	49	22	66	30
8	46	117	50	126	54	136	44	20	55	25	77	35
9	48	122	52	132	56	143	49	22	62	28	90	41
10	50	127	54	138	59	149	53	24	73	33	104	47
11	52	133	57	144	61	156	60	27	82	37	119	54
12	55	140	59	151	64	163	66	30	93	42	134	61
13	57	145	62	157	66	168	75	34	101	46	148	67
14	59	149	63	160	67	171	84	38	110	50	161	73
15	59	150	64	162	68	173	90	41	119	54	172	78
16	59	151	64	163	68	173	95	43	123	56	179	81
17	60	153	64	163	69	174	97	44	126	57	209	95
18	61	154	65	164	69	174	99	45	126	57	209	95

SOURCE: Based on data from National Center for Health Statistics: NCHS Growth Charts, Health Resources Administration, Rockville, Maryland, 1976.

various heights and body build. Height and weight data for boys and girls between 2 and 18 years of age is also provided for general information (Tables 4.3 and 4.4). A weight that is 10 percent above the desirable weight in the normal individual is considered overweight and 20 percent above the desirable weight is indicative of obesity. Obesity is accompanied by increase in fat or adipose tissue. Increase of the fat tissue is dependent upon the number (hyperplasia) and size (hypertrophy) of the fat cells (adipocytes), both of which are influenced by variables such as diet and heredity. The early-onset or childhood obesity is frequently accompanied by an increase in the number of fat cells, whereas adult-onset obesity is more commonly accompanied by increase in size of fat cells. Studies on adipose tissue or fat cells have led to the following conclusions:

1. Adults, whether normal or obese, have a fixed number of fat cells in the body, therefore, obesity developing in adult life is associated only with the enlargement of fat cells.
2. Obesity developing in infancy or childhood is associated with an increase in cell number. The infant-feeding practices which involve high energy intakes, stimulate an increase in the number of fat cells.
3. Obesity caused by an increase in the number of fat cells is more resistant to weight-reduction treatment than an increase in size of fat cells.

4. The size of the fat cell influences its metabolism. For example, increased insulin resistance in large cells leads to an increase in insulin requirements and a tendency to develop diabetes.

At least one practical lesson is obvious from the above conclusions—that childhood nutrition does apparently effect fat cell numbers. Therefore, it is important to introduce youngsters to good eating habits which are nutritionally sound but avoid excessive fat consumption or other excessively high calorie diets. In this way, it is possible to prevent a tendency towards obesity in later life. Higher consumption of carefully selected natural foods as emphasized in Chapter 5 is one way to introduce children to sound eating habits, which should last a life time. (The lack of exercise does not cause overweight, even though it is important for physical fitness, and has an indirect effect on weight through expending more calories.)

Being too fat and being overweight may not always be the same. Heavy bones and muscles can make a person overweight in terms of the charts, but only an excess amount of fat tissue can make someone obese. Although height and weight tables are generally used to determine obesity (e.g. Tables 4.1 and 4.2), another method which can be useful to estimate an excess amount of fat is the "pinch" test. The thickness of the fat located directly under the skin can be measured at places such as the back of the upper arm, directly under the shoulder blade or around the waist. The measurement can be performed either by skinfold calipers or simply by pinching the fold between the fingers. If pinched thickness is more than one inch at any of the areas, the likelihood is that the person is obese.

What Causes Overweight

Overweight or obesity is generally accepted to be the result of energy intake that is greater than energy expended. In other words, excess weight is the result of an imbalance between energy (measured in calories) consumed as food and energy expended, either in maintaining the basic metabolic processes necessary to sustain life or in performing physical activity. The calories consumed in excess of their use become converted to fat and accumulate in the body as fat, or adipose tissue. It is believed that the rate of fat deposition is higher in overweight people as compared to those with normal weight (due to the effect of overweight on body physiology). Factors which influence obesity and upset the caloric balance may include heredity, endocrine factors, physical activity of an individual, number of fat cells, greater intestinal length, or psychosocial-emotional problems. In the psychosocial aspects of over-eating, people experience frustration, depression, worry, guilt, shame, hopelessness, isolation and unusual stress which often leads them to seek compensation in eating. To prevent an increase in body weight and body fat because of a caloric imbalance, any program of weight control must establish an equilibrium between energy input and energy output. If you consume more calories than you use—whether from protein, carbohydrate, or fat—you will gain weight. And if you consume fewer calories than you use—you will lose body fat.

Weight and Mortality

Vital statistics show that thin people live longer than those who are overweight (see Table 4.5). A moderate degree of underweight is advantageous. Consequently,

Table 4.5 **Mortality of men in different weight classes.**

| Weight Class | | Percent decrease or increase over normal death rate* | | | | | |
| | | Ages under 40 | | | Ages 40 and over | | |
		Short men	Medium men	Tall men	Short men	Medium men	Tall men
Underweight:							
40 lb below	(18 kg) average	15	15	—	20	0	0
20 lb below	(9 kg) average	−5	−10	−10	0	−5	−5
Average weight:		0	0	0	0	0	0
Overweight:							
20 lb above	(9 kg) average	15	10	10	20	20	10
40 lb above	(18 kg) average	35	25	25	35	30	25
60 lb above	(27 kg) average	90	45	45	60	50	45

*For example, 20 1b above average weight for short men under age 40 increase chances of death by 15%, whereas 20 1b below average decrease by 5% over normal death rate.

SOURCE: Based on 1959 Build and Blood Pressure Study, Society of Actuaries, Chicago.

those who wish a long and healthy life should keep their weight slightly below, rather than at, the average level for age, height, and body build (see Tables 4.1 and 4.2). Overweight, on the other hand, is disadvantageous, with excess mortality roughly proportional to the degree of overweight. Only 60 percent of obese people (20% or more overweight) reach the age of 60, compared with 90 percent of slim persons. Thirty percent of the obese reach the age of 70, while 50 percent of the slim reach 70. The age of 80 is reached by only 10 percent of the obese, compared with 30 percent of the thin, a ratio of one to three. The effects of overweight on mortality show that overweight is associated with excessive mortality from heart disease, diabetes, nephritis, cerebral hemorrhage, and various diseases of the digestive system. Overweight people have difficulties with their feet and back because of the added burden of weight on the skeleton, and have, as well an increased incidence of gout and arthritis. They suffer from shortness of breath, especially on exertion and face increased risk of surgery.

A Calorie

A Calorie is the unit used for measuring the heat or energy producing value of food when it is burned by the body. One Calorie produces enough heart to raise the temperature of 1 kilogram of water one degree centigrade (from 14.5° to 15.5°C); in human nutrition it is more often used as kilocalorie (abbreviated kcal). In this book we will use the word "Calorie," which is more familiar to most of us. In the diet, a calorie describes the amount of energy potentially available in a given food. It is also used to describe the amount of energy the body must use up to perform a given function. The International Organization for Standardization (ISC) recommends the adoption of the *Joule* as the preferred unit for energy measurements in all branches of science. The nutritional Calorie is a measure of thermal (heat) energy and the Joule is a measure of mechanical energy. To convert Calories to Joules, one multiplies Calories by 4.184. For example, the value of 4 Calories per gram of carbohydrate converted to Joules will be (4×4.184) or approximately 17 Joules per gram. The American Institute of Nutrition in 1970 recommended that replacement of the Calories by Joules be effected as soon as the mechanics of the transition can be established.

Caloric Value of Foods

The total caloric content (total energy) of a food can be measured by means of a device called a bomb calorimeter, where the rise in temperature of the water after the burning of food in an oxygen atmosphere can be used to calculate the heat energy of calories generated. The caloric value of a specific food depends on the composition of the food in terms of protein, fat and carbohydrate. The amount of heat produced per 100 gram (3.5 ounce or 1/2 cup) of purified protein, carbohydrate and fat is 565, 410 and 945 Calories, respectively (see Table 4.6). In the body some of the food is not completely digested, and the extent to which the ingested nutrients are available to the cells, or their digestibility, is of importance. Normally about 98 percent of the carbohydrate, 95 percent of the fat and 92 percent of the protein is absorbed and thus provides digestible energy. As far as utilization by the cell is concerned, carbohydrate and fat are completely oxidized and their calorie yield is the same as for digestible energy. The amino (NH_2) group of protein amino acids is not completely oxidized, but is excreted in the urine, chiefly as urea, with smaller amounts of creatinine, uric acid and other compounds; therefore available energy to the cell from protein is less than digestible energy (see Table 4.6). When the average efficiency of digestion is taken into account, the net caloric value for protein, carbohydrate, and fat are 400 Calories per 100 gram of protein as well as carbohydrate, and 900 Calories per 100 gram of fat. For all practical purposes, to estimate the caloric values of food, 1 gram of protein contains 4 Calories, as does 1 gram of carbohydrate. One gram of fat, by contrast, contains 9 Calories. Because most foods in the normal diet consist of various proportions of these three nutrients, the caloric value of a given

Table 4.6   Energy values in Calories per 100 g (3.5 ounces) of purified protein, carbohydrate and fat.

Source of Food Energy	Gross Energy of Food	Digestible Energy (after subtracting energy in feces)	Metabolizable (Available) Energy (after subtracting energy in urine)
Protein	565	520	400
Carbohydrate	410	400	400
Fat	945	900	900

SOURCE: Pike, R.L. and M.L. Brown. *Nutrition: An integrated approach*, 2nd ed. John Wiley and Sons, 1975.

food is determined by the amount of protein, carbohydrate and fat. For example, the caloric value of 2 eggs of known nutrient composition weighing 100 g can be calculated as follows:

	Percent	Total grams	Calories
Protein	13%	13 g	$13 \times 4 = 52$
Carbohydrate	1%	1 g	$1 \times 4 = 4$
Fat	12%	12 g	$12 \times 9 = 108$
	Total Calories for 2 eggs weighing 100 g		$= 164$

To calculate the caloric content of liquor, the following equation can be used:
  0.8 Cal./proof/ounce
For example, to calculate the caloric content of 2 ounce-80 proof scotch:
  $0.8 \times 80 \times 2 = 128$ Calories

The caloric values of common foods are given in Table 4.7. The table also provides percentages of total calories of fat, protein and carbohydrate for each of the listed foods. This is useful for a quick glance at the nutritive value of foods in addition to their caloric values. However, the foods consumed as extra calories are always converted to fat and accumulate in the body as fat, no matter what the ratio of protein, carbohydrate and fat. Therefore, avoiding the excessive caloric intake is most important for good health and proper weight.

Determining Proper Calorie Intake

A certain number of calories is needed each day to maintain a constant weight. Decide on your ideal weight with the help of Tables 4.1 and 4.2. If you are moderately active, multiply your ideal weight by 15. If you are very active by 20. For example—if you are a moderately active, 150-pounder, you need $= 150 \times 15 = 2,250$ Calories/day; if you are a very active, 150-pounder, you need $= 150 \times 20 = 3,000$ Calories/day. Although this is a crude method, it is accurate enough for

Table 4.7   Caloric values of common foods and percent of total calories of protein, carbohydrate and fat.

Food	Approx. measure	Weight (grams)	Total cal	% Protein cal	% Carbo-hydrate cal	% Fat cal
MILK AND MILK PRODUCTS						
Milk:						
Fluid:						
Whole (3.5% fat)	1 cup	244	160	22	29	49
Nonfat (skim)	1 cup	245	90	43	56	Trace
Partly skimmed (2% fat)	1 cup	246	145	28	41	31
Dry, nonfat instant:						
Low-density (1 1/3 cups needed for reconstitution to 1 qt.)	1 cup	68	245	41	58	Trace
High-density (7/8 cup needed for reconstitution to 1 qt.)	1 cup	104	375	40	58	2
Cheese:						
Blue or Roquefort	1 oz	28	105	25	2	73
Cheddar	1 oz	28	115	27	2	71
Cottage, large or small curd:						
creamed	1 oz	28	30	55	11	35
Uncreamed	1 oz	28	24	84	12	3
Parmesan grated	1 oz	28	130	39	3	58
Swiss	1 oz	28	105	32	2	67
Pasteurized processed cheese:						
American	1 oz	28	105	25	3	72
Cream:						
Half-and-half (cream and milk)	1 cup	242	325	10	13	77
Sour cream	1 cup	230	485	7	10	83
Whipped topping (pressurized)	1 cup	60	155	5	15	80
Butter	3.5 oz	100	716	Trace	Trace	99
Milk beverages:						
Cocoa, homemade	1 cup	250	245	16	42	42
Malted milk	1 cup	235	245	18	45	37
Milk desserts:						
Ice cream						
Regular (approx. 10% fat)	1 cup	133	255	9	43	48

Table 4.7 continued

Food	Approx. measure	Weight (grams)	Total cal	% Protein cal	% Carbo- hydrate cal	% Fat cal
Yoghurt:						
Made from partially skimmed milk	1 cup	245	125	27	43	30
Made from whole milk	1 cup	245	150	19	32	49
EGGS						
Large whole, without shell	1 egg	50	80	34	2	64
White of egg	1 white	33	15	93	6	Trace
Yolk of egg	1 yolk	17	60	20	1	79
MEAT						
Bacon, (20 slices per lb. raw), broiled or fried, crisp	2 slices	15	90	21	4	75
Hamburger (ground beef), broiled Lean	3 ounces	85	185	51	0	49
Regular (ground beef) broiled	3 ounces	85	245	35	0	65
Steak, broiled:						
Relatively, fat, such as sirloin:						
Lean and fat	3 ounces	85	330	25	0	75
Lean only	3 ounces	85	173	67	0	33
Relatively, lean, such as round:						
Lean and fat	3 ounces	85	220	45	0	55
Lean only	3 ounces	85	163	70	0	30
Corned beef	3 ounces	85	185	49	0	51
Beef and vegetable stew	1 cup	235	210	29	28	43
Chilli con carne, canned:						
With beans	1 cup	250	335	23	36	41
Without beans	1 cup	255	510	21	12	67
Bologna, slice, 3-in diam. by 1/8 inch.	2 slices	26	80	16	Trace	84
Frankfurter, heated (8 per lb. purchased pkg.)	1 frank	56	170	17	2	81
Salami, cooked	1 oz	28	90	24	Trace	76
Chicken						
All classes:						
Light meat without skin, raw	3.5 oz	100	117	85	0	15
Light meat without skin, cooked	3.5 oz	100	166	81	0	18

Table 4.7 continued

Food	Approx. measure	Weight (grams)	Total cal	% Protein cal	% Carbo-hydrate cal	% Fat cal
Dark meat without skin, raw	3.5 oz	100	130	68	0	33
Dark meat without skin, cooked	3.5 oz	100	176	68	0	32
Chicken:						
Roasters:						
Light meat without skin, cooked	3.5 oz	100	182	76	0	24
Dark meat without skin, cooked	3.5 oz	100	184	68	0	32
Fryers:						
Light meat without skin, raw	3.5 oz	100	101	87	0	13
Breast, raw	3.5 oz	100	110	81	0	20
Thigh, raw	3.5 oz	100	128	60	0	39
Turkey:						
Flesh only, all classes, cooked	3.5 oz	100	190	71	0	29
Light meat, all classes, cooked	3.5 oz	100	176	80	0	20
Dark meat, all classes, cooked	3.5 oz	100	203	63	0	37
Duck:						
Domesticated, flesh only, raw	3.5 oz	100	165	49	0	55
Wild, flesh only, raw	3.5 oz	100	138	34	0	66
Squab:						
Light meat without skin, raw	3.5 oz	100	125	70	0	30
Fish and Shellfish:						
Fish						
Barracuda, pacific, raw	3.5 oz	100	113	79	0	21
Bass:						
Black sea, raw	3.5 oz	100	93	88	0	12
Striped, raw	3.5 oz	100	105	77	0	23
White, raw	3.5 oz	100	98	78	0	21
Carp, raw	3.5 oz	100	115	67	0	33
Catfish, raw	3.5 oz	100	103	73	0	27
Cod						
raw	3.5 oz	100	78	96	0	3
canned	3.5 oz	100	85	96	0	3

Table 4.7 continued

Food	Approx. measure	Weight (grams)	Total cal	% Protein cal	% Carbo-hydrate cal	% Fat cal
Flatfishes (flounders, soles, sanddabs), raw	3.5 oz	100	79	90	0	9
Haddock, raw	3.5 oz	100	79	99	0	1
Halibut:						
Atlantic and Pacific, raw	3.5 oz	100	100	89	0	11
California, raw	3.5 oz	100	97	87	0	13
Herring:						
Atlantic, raw	3.5 oz	100	176	42	0	58
Pacific, raw	3.5 oz	100	98	76	0	24
Mackerel:						
Atlantic, raw	3.5 oz	100	191	42	0	58
Pacific, raw	3.5 oz	100	159	41	0	59
Ocean perch:						
Atlantic, raw	3.5 oz	100	88	87	0	12
Pacific, raw	3.5 oz	100	95	85	0	14
Perch						
White, raw	3.5 oz	100	118	70	0	31
Yellow, raw	3.5 oz	100	91	91	0	9
Pike:						
Blue, raw	3.5 oz	100	90	91	0	9
Northern, raw	3.5 oz	100	88	89	0	11
Walleye, raw	3.5 oz	100	93	89	0	12
Pompano, raw	3.5 oz	100	166	48	0	52
Salmon:						
Atlantic, raw	3.5 oz	100	217	44	0	56
Chinook, raw	3.5 oz	100	222	37	0	67
Atlantic, canned, solids and liquids	3.5 oz	100	203	46	0	54
Chinook, canned, solids and liquids	3.5 oz	100	210	40	0	60
Sockeye, canned, solids and liquids	3.5 oz	100	171	51	0	49
Seabass, white, raw	3.5 oz	100	96	95	0	5
Snapper, red and gray, raw	3.5 oz	100	93	91	0	9
Sturgeon:						
Raw	3.5 oz	100	94	82	0	18
Cooked, steamed	3.5 oz	100	160	68	0	32
Swordfish, raw	3.5 oz	100	118	69	0	31
Trout:						
Brook, raw	3.5 oz	100	101	81	0	19

Table 4.7 continued

Food	Approx. measure	Weight (grams)	Total cal	% Protein cal	% Carbo- hydrate cal	% Fat cal
Rainbow (steelhead), raw	3.5 oz	100	195	47	0	53
Tuna:						
Bluefin, raw	3.5 oz	100	145	74	0	26
Yellowfin, raw	3.5 oz	100	133	79	0	20
Canned in water, solids and liquids	3.5 oz	100	127	94	0	6
Whitefish, lake, raw	3.5 oz	100	155	52	0	48
Yellowtail (Pacific coast), raw	3.5 oz	100	138	65	0	35
Shellfish:						
Abalone, raw	3.5 oz	100	98	81	14	5
Clams:						
Soft, meat only, raw	3.5 oz	100	82	73	6	21
Hard, meat only, raw	3.5 oz	100	80	59	30	10
Mixed, canned, drained solids	3.5 oz	100	98	69	8	23
Mixed, canned, liquor	3.5 oz	100	19	52	45	5
Crab:						
Steamed	3.5 oz	100	93	79	2	18
Canned	3.5 oz	100	101	74	4	22
Lobster, northern						
Whole, raw	3.5 oz	100	91	79	2	19
Canned, or cooked	3.5 oz	100	95	84	1	14
Mussels, Atlantic and Pacific, meat only, raw	3.5 oz	100	95	65	14	21
Oysters:						
Eastern, meat only, raw	3.5 oz	100	66	54	21	25
Pacific and western, meat only, raw	3.5 oz	100	91	50	29	22
Canned, solids and liquids	3.5 oz	100	76	48	26	26
Scallops:						
Raw	3.5 oz	100	81	81	17	2
Cooked, steamed	3.5 oz	100	112	88	0	11
Shrimp:						
Raw	3.5 oz	100	91	85	7	8
Canned, drained solids	3.5 oz	100	116	89	2	9

Table 4.7 continued

Food	Approx. measure	Weight (grams)	Total cal	% Protein cal	% Carbo-hydrate cal	% Fat cal
CEREAL GRAINS						
Grains:						
Barley, pearled (light), raw	3.5 oz	100	349	8	89	2
Buckwheat:						
Whole-grain (kasha), raw	3.5 oz	100	335	12	82	6
Flour, dark	3.5 oz	100	333	12	82	6
Cornmeal, white or yellow:						
Whole ground, unbolted	3.5 oz	100	355	7	84	9
Oatmeal (rolled oats):						
Dry	3.5 oz	100	390	13	72	16
Cooked	3.5 oz	100	55	13	73	15
Popcorn:						
Unpopped	3.5 oz	100	362	9	80	11
Popped, plain	3.5 oz	100	386	9	80	11
Rice:						
Brown, raw	3.5 oz	100	360	7	89	4
Brown, cooked	3.5 oz	100	119	7	88	4
White, raw	3.5 oz	100	363	7	92	1
White, cooked	3.5 oz	100	109	7	92	1
Rye:						
Whole-grain, raw	3.5 oz	100	334	11	85	4
Flour, medium	3.5 oz	100	350	11	85	4
Wheat:						
Bulgar (parboiled whole wheat), variety average, dry	3.5 oz	100	356	10	82	3
Whole-grain, variety average, raw	3.5 oz	100	330	13	81	5
Flour, whole (from hard wheats)	3.5 oz	100	333	14	81	5
Flour, white all-purpose (patent)	3.5 oz	100	364	12	86	2
DRIED LEGUMES						
Black, brown, bayo beans, raw	3.5 oz	100	339	23	74	4
Chickpeas or gar-banzos, raw	3.5 oz	100	360	20	69	11

Table 4.7 continued

Food	Approx. measure	Weight (grams)	Total cal	% Protein cal	% Carbo-hydrate cal	% Fat cal
Lentils:						
Whole, raw	3.5 oz	100	340	25	72	3
Whole, cooked	3.5 oz	100	106	26	74	Trace
Split without seed coat, raw	3.5 oz	100	345	25	74	2
Lima beans:						
Raw	3.5 oz	100	345	20	75	4
Cooked	3.5 oz	100	138	20	75	4
Peanuts:						
Raw, with skins	3.5 oz	100	564	16	13	70
Roasted, with skins	3.5 oz	100	582	16	14	70
Peanut butter (without sweetener)	3.5 oz	100	581	17	12	71
Peas, split:						
Raw	3.5 oz	100	348	24	73	2
Cooked	3.5 oz	100	115	24	74	2
Pinto, calico, red Mexican beans, raw	3.5 oz	100	349	23	74	3
Soybeans:						
Raw	3.5 oz	100	403	29	34	37
Cooked	3.5 oz	100	130	29	34	37
NUT, SEEDS						
Almonds	3.5 oz	100	598	11	13	76
Brazil nuts	3.5 oz	100	654	7	7	86
Cashews	3.5 oz	100	561	11	21	68
Chestnuts:						
Fresh	3.5 oz	100	194	5	88	6
Dried	3.5 oz	100	377	6	85	9
Coconut:						
Meat, fresh	3.5 oz	100	346	3	11	85
Meat, dried, unsweetened	3.5 oz	100	662	4	14	82
Filberts (hazelnuts)	3.5 oz	100	634	7	11	82
Macadamias	3.5 oz	100	691	4	9	87
Peanuts, see "Dried Legumes"						
Pecans	3.5 oz	100	687	5	9	87
Sesame seeds, dried	3.5 oz	100	582	11	12	77
Sunflower seed kernels, dried	3.5 oz	100	560	15	14	71
Walnuts, English or Persian	3.5 oz	100	651	8	10	82

Table 4.7 continued

Food	Approx. measure	Weight (grams)	Total cal	% Protein cal	% Carbo-hydrate cal	% Fat cal
VEGETABLES						
Artichokes, globe or French, cooked	3.5 oz	100	44	15	80	4
Asparagus, cooked	3.5 oz	100	20	27	64	8
Avocados, raw	1 Avocado	284	370	4	13	82
Bamboo shoots, raw	3.5 oz	100	27	23	69	9
Beans:						
limas, cooked	3.5 oz	100	111	24	72	4
snap green, cooked	3.5 oz	100	25	16	77	7
yellow or wax, cooked	3.5 oz	100	22	16	76	8
Bean sprouts (mung beans), raw	3.5 oz	100	35	27	68	5
Beets, red, cooked (2 beets, 2-inch diam)	3.5 oz	100	32	10	86	3
Broccoli, raw	3.5 oz	100	32	27	66	8
Brussels sprouts, cooked	3.5 oz	100	36	28	63	9
Cabbage, raw	3.5 oz	100	24	13	80	7
Carrots, raw (5.5 by 1 inch).	1 carrot	50	20	7	89	4
Cauliflower, raw	3.5 oz	100	27	24	69	6
Celery, raw	3.5 oz	100	17	13	82	5
Chives, raw	3.5 oz	100	28	16	74	9
Collards, cooked	3.5 oz	100	29	23	60	17
Corn kernels, sweet, cooked (approximate values)	3.5 oz	100	83	9	81	9
Cucumbers:						
pared, raw, 7½ by 2 inch	1 cucumber	200	28	10	83	6
unpared, raw, 7½ by 2 inch	1 cucumber	207	30	14	80	5
Eggplant, cooked	3.5 oz	100	19	13	78	9
Endive, curly and escarole, raw	3.5 oz	100	20	21	74	4
Garlic cloves, raw	3.5 oz	100	137	12	86	1
Kale, cooked	3.5 oz	100	28	28	51	21
Leeks, raw	3.5 oz	100	52	12	83	5

Table 4.7 continued

Food	Approx. measure	Weight (grams)	Total cal	% Protein cal	% Carbo-hydrate cal	% Fat cal
Lettuce:						
Butterhead varieties, e.g.,						
Bibb, raw, 4-inch diameter	1 head	220	30	22	66	12
Crisphead varieties, e.g.,						
iceberg, raw 4.75-inch diameter	1 head	454	60	16	78	6
Romaine, or cos, raw	3.5 oz	100	18	18	69	14
Mushrooms, raw	3.5 oz	100	28	25	55	9
Mustard greens, cooked	3.5 oz	100	23	23	62	14
Okra, cooked	3.5 oz	100	29	17	74	9
Olives, ripe, canned	3.5 oz	100	129	3	7	90
Onions, mature, raw, 2.5 inch, diameter	1 onion	110	40	11	88	2
Onions, green, raw	3.5 oz	100	36	10	84	5
Parsley, raw	3.5 oz	100	44	20	69	11
Parsnips, cooked	3.5 oz	100	66	6	87	6
Peas, edible-podded, raw	3.5 oz	100	53	16	81	3
Peas, green, cooked	3.5 oz	100	71	26	69	5
Peppers, bell raw	3.5 oz	100	22	13	78	8
Potatoes, baked in skin	3.5 oz	100	93	8	91	1
Potatoes, boiled in skin	3.5 oz	100	76	8	91	1
Pumpkin, canned	3.5 oz	100	33	7	85	7
Radishes, raw, small	1 radish	10	1.5	16	80	5
Rutabagas, cooked	3.5 oz	100	35	7	90	2
Spinach, cooked	3.5 oz	100	23	32	56	11
Squash, summer, cooked	3.5 oz	100	14	16	78	6
Squash, winter, cooked, baked	3.5 oz	100	63	7	88	5
Sweet potatoes, cooked, baked in skim milk	3.5 oz	100	141	4	93	3
Swisschard, cooked	3.5 oz	100	18	25	66	9
Tapioca, dry	3.5 oz	100	352	0.5	99	0.5

Table 4.7 continued

Food	Approx. measure	Weight (grams)	Total cal	% Protein cal	% Carbo-hydrate cal	% Fat cal
Tomatoes, ripe, raw, 3 inch diameter	1 tomato	200	40	12	76	8
Tomato juice, canned or bottled	3.5 oz	100	19	12	81	4
Turnips, cooked	3.5 oz	100	23	10	83	7
Water chestnut, raw	3.5 oz	100	79	5	94	2
Watercress, raw	3.5 oz	100	19	29	57	13
Zucchini, see Squash, summer	3.5 oz	100	14	16	78	6
FRUITS						
Apples, raw	1 apple	150	70	1	90	9
Apple juice, canned or bottled	3.5 oz	100	47	1	99	Trace
Apricots, raw, 1 medium	1 apricot	38	18	7	90	3
Bananas, raw, 1 medium	1 banana	175	100	4	94	2
Blackberries (incl. boysenberries) raw	3.5 oz	100	58	7	80	13
Blueberries, raw	3.5 oz	100	62	4	89	7
Breadfruit, raw	3.5 oz	100	103	6	92	2
Cantaloupe, see Muskmelons						
Casaba melon, see Muskmelons						
Cherries:						
Sour red, raw	3.5 oz	100	58	7	88	4
Sweet, raw	3.5 oz	100	70	6	90	4
Cranberries, raw	3.5 oz	100	46	3	84	13
Dates, dried	3.5 oz	100	274	3	96	1
Figs:						
Raw	3.5 oz	100	80	5	92	3
Dried	3.5 oz	100	274	5	91	4
Gooseberries, raw	3.5 oz	100	39	7	89	4
Grapefruit, raw	3.5 oz	100	41	4	93	2
Granadilla, raw	3.5 oz	100	90	8	85	6
Grapes:						
Slip skin (incl. Concord), raw	3.5 oz	100	69	6	82	12
Adherent skin (incl. Thompson seed-less, muscat), raw	3.5 oz	100	67	3	93	4
Guava, raw	3.5 oz	100	62	4	87	8

Table 4.7 continued

Food	Approx. measure	Weight (grams)	Total cal	% Protein cal	% Carbo-hydrate cal	% Fat cal
Kumquats, raw	3.5 oz	100	65	5	94	1
Lemon juice	3.5 oz	100	25	7	86	7
Loganberries, raw	3.5 oz	100	62	3	94	3
Lychees, raw	3.5 oz	100	48	5	92	4
Mangos, raw	3.5 oz	100	64	5	92	4
Muskmelons:						
Cantaloupe, raw	3.5 oz	100	30	8	90	3
Casaba, raw	3.5 oz	100	27	15	87	Trace
Honeydew, raw	3.5 oz	100	33	8	84	8
Nectarines, raw	3.5 oz	100	64	3	96	Trace
Oranges, raw	1 orange	180	65	7	90	3
Orange juice	3.5 oz	100	45	5	91	4
Papayas, raw	3.5 oz	100	39	5	92	2
Peaches, raw	1 peach	114	35	5	92	2
Pears, raw	1 pear	182	100	2	95	3
Persimmons, raw	3.5 oz	100	127	4	90	5
Pineapple, raw	3.5 oz	100	52	3	95	3
Plums, raw	1 plum	60	25	2	97	Trace
Pomegranates, raw	3.5 oz	100	63	3	94	4
Quinces, raw	3.5 oz	100	57	2	97	1
Raisins, natural, uncooked	3.5 oz	100	289	3	96	1
Raspberries, red, raw	3.5 oz	100	57	7	86	7
Strawberries, raw	3.5 oz	100	37	6	82	11
Tangerines, raw, medium	1 tangerine	116	40	6	91	4
Watermelon, raw	3.5 oz	100	26	6	87	6
FATS, OIL:						
Oils, salad or cooking	3.5 oz	100	884	0	0	100
Margarine	3.5 oz	100	720	Trace	Trace	99
SUGARS, SWEETS:						
Cake icings:						
Chocolate made with milk and table fat.	1 cup	275	1,035	3	66	31
Coconut (with boiled icing).	1 cup	166	605	2	79	19
Creamy fudge from mix with water only	1 cup	245	830	3	81	16
White, boiled	1 cup	94	300	1	99	0
Candy:						
Caramels, plain or chocolate.	1 oz	28	115	3	74	23

Table 4.7 continued

Food	Approx. measure	Weight (grams)	Total cal	% Protein cal	% Carbo-hydrate cal	% Fat cal
Chocolate, milk, plain	1 oz	28	145	5	42	53
Chocolate-coated peanuts	1 oz	28	160	11	26	63
Gum drops	1 oz	28	100	Trace	100	Trace
Marshmallows	1 oz	28	90	4	96	Trace
Sugars:						
Brown, firm packed	1 cup	220	820	0	109	0
White, granulated	1 cup	200	770	0	109	0
	1 tbsp	11	40	0	100	0
BEVERAGES:						
Beverages, alcoholic:						
Beer	12 fl. oz	360	150	3	37	0
Gin, rum, vodka, whiskey:						
80-proof	1½ fl. oz jigger	42	100	0	Trace	0
86-proof	1½ fl. oz jigger	42	105	0	Trace	0
90-proof	1½ fl. oz jigger	42	110	0	Trace	0
94-proof	1½ fl. oz jigger	42	115	0	Trace	0
100-proof	1½ fl. oz jigger	42	125	0	Trace	0
Brandy, or cognac	1 brandy glass (1 oz)	30	75	0	Trace	0
Wines:						
Dessert	3½ fl. oz glass	103	140	Trace	23	0
Table	3½ fl. oz glass	102	85	Trace	19	0
Champagne	3½ fl. oz glass	120	85	Trace	14	0
Vermouth, sweet	3½ fl. oz glass	100	170	Trace	28	0
Vermouth, dry	3½ fl. oz glass	100	105	Trace	4	0
Cola type	12 fl. oz	369	145	0	100	0
Ginger ale	12 fl. oz	366	115	0	100	0
Root beer	12 fl. oz	370	150	0	100	0
Gelatin dessert, prepared with water	1 cup	240	140	11	89	0

SOURCE: Values mainly based on U. S. Department of Agriculture Handbook No. 8.

many purposes. The crudeness of this method is due to the fact that no correction is made for sex or age, and the estimation of activity is a rough one. Table 4.8 lists the daily calorie-requirements for various subjects. Make an important note of the decrease in calorie requirement with increased age in adults. In general, calorie requirement for individuals over 50 years of age should be reduced to 90 percent of the amount required by a mature adult. For example, a person consuming 3,000 Calories would need to reduce his intake to about 2,700 Calories. (For further information on setting a calorie limit, see section, "The Calorie-restricted Diet Plan" in this Chapter.)

Table 4.8   Daily dietary allowances for calories.[1]

Subjects	Age[2] (years)	Weight (kg)	Weight (lb)	Height (cm)	Height (in)	Calories
Men	25	70	154	175	69	3,200
	45	70	154	175	69	3,000
	65	70	154	175	69	2,550
Women[3]	25	58	128	163	64	2,330
	45	58	128	163	64	2,200
	65	58	128	163	64	1,800
Infants	0 to 1/12	—	—	—	—	—
	2/12 to 6/12	6	13	60	24	kg × 120
	7/12 to 12/12	9	20	70	28	kg × 100
Children	1 to 3	12	27	87	34	1,300
	4 to 6	18	40	109	43	1,700
	10 to 12	36	79	144	57	2,500
Boys	13 to 15	49	108	163	64	3,100
	16 to 19	63	139	175	69	3,600
Girls	13 to 15	49	108	160	63	2,600
	16 to 19	54	120	163	64	2,400

[1]Allowances for normally active persons in a temperate climate.
[2]Note decrease in calorie requirement with increasing age for adults.
[3]A woman in the second half of pregnancy should have +300 Calories daily. A woman with a daily lactation of 850 ml should have +1,000 Calories.
SOURCE: Food and Nutrition Board, National Research Council, 1958.

Treatment of Overweight

It is only when the number of calories ingested as food exceeds the daily energy requirements that the excess calories are stored as fat in adipose tissue. Therefore, regardless of the cause of overweight (such as genetic make up or poor eating habits), there are two ways to lose weight: (a) either cut down food calories taken in (the dietary control of weight), or (b) raise the number of calories expended as energy, through physical activity.

As you may have noticed, many popular books or articles on exotic diets or exercise plans usually claim their plans to be easy and effortless to follow. If this were the case, then millions of adults and teenagers who are overweight could be cured easily. Generally the exotic diets produce a weight loss primarily due to loss of body water during the first several weeks. Unless a person can maintain a reduced caloric intake for a considerable time, the weight will eventually be regained. The net result is a return to original body size, often at the expense of feelings of hunger and other psychological stresses while the diet plan is actually followed. In fact, people who live from one best-selling weight-loss scheme to the next, often end up with rhythmic, loss and gain patterns of weight. Studies indicate that the repeated gaining, losing, and regaining of extra pounds is more damaging to physical health than just remaining overweight. That's why it's so important to forget all the gimmicks—the crash programs and diets you could not possibly follow for long—and find instead a permanent solution to your weight problem.

A review of the scientific literature dealing with weight loss in obese subjects reveals that people who are initially successful in modifying their body composition are usually unsuccessful in permanently maintaining their desired body size and shape. Such statistics indicate that the long-term maintenance of a particular low-calorie diet is extremely difficult. Similarly, increasing energy expenditure through physical activity, while not unpleasant in itself, does require a personal commitment in terms of time and life style that many people are not willing to make.

Some of the common weight loss practices are discussed in this Chapter, which are effective only to a certain degree for various lengths of time, many of these at the cost of a physical as well as psychological health loss. The permanent and painless solution to an overweight problem is a change of eating habits that requires health awareness, and the adoption of a natural diet as discussed in detail in Chapter 5. The natural diet is not even a diet plan and no emphasis is placed on counting the calories. It simply suggests a variety of whole natural health foods (menus included as Appendix) low in calories and saturated fat but high in health-promoting minerals and vitamins. Since these are in fact health foods rather than diet foods, they cause no risk of complications such as malnutrition which often accompany less well-founded crash diets.

The Dietary Control of Weight: Regulation of food intake is an effective means of controlling body weight. The principle involved is simply that of keeping the energy intake equal to the energy expenditure of the body. When the energy value of food eaten is less than the energy expenditure, stored body fat is called upon to make up the deficit, and weight is consequently lost.

Fad Diets: Periodically, new diets for weight reduction become popular. Some of these may be followed effectively and safely for short periods, whereas others are nutritionally inadequate and should be avoided. Most of the fad diets which frequently reappear under various names (*The Scarsdale Diet, Atkins' Diet, Dr. Stillman's Diet*) contain no- or low-carbohydrate, highprotein, moderate- or high-fat. Since these diets are high in fat and low in carbohydrates, the free blood sugar (glucose) is rapidly burned off, forcing the body to depend on its fat reserves for energy. The fatty acids derived from the fat reserve burn inefficiently and produce acid metabolites called ketones. The abnormal increase of ketones is called *ketosis*. Therefore, the diet is meant to put the dieter into a state of ketosis, which supposedly increases the rate of weight loss and may reduce hunger. There is another fad diet called *Starch Blockers* that also put the dieter in a state of ketosis. The diet tablets block the action of enzyme that helps in starch digestion. Therefore, body cannot use starch calories from foods and use only fat and protein calories. In itself, the high fat diet designed to put the dieter in a state of ketosis is accompanied by serious complications. For example, the brain is partially starved by the absence of glucose and loses its efficiency. Ketones being acid metabolites change the pH of blood. If the blood becomes acidic enough, one can go into ketosis shock which may sometimes be fatal. Moreover, acidic blood does impair proper functioning of body and brain, thus affecting both physical and mental performance.

The danger of fad diets being nutritionally unbalanced in one way or another is a real hazard even to a healthy person. For example, the popular Atkins low-carbohydrate diet cause deficiencies in calcium, vitamins A and C, thiamin, riboflavin, and niacin because it excludes bread and cereal products and drastically limits servings of fruits and vegetables and milk products (except fat-laden cheese). At the same time, it's loaded with protein, saturated animal fats, and cholesterol: bacon, eggs, sausages, cheese, roast beef, steak, fried chicken—a heart attack's delight. Like the one above, most such diets are high in saturated animal fats and cholesterol, which can raise the blood levels of cholesterol, and speed the development of atherosclerosis, the leading cause of premature death in the United States.

The followers of many of these diets do lose weight rapidly during the first week or so because of fluid loss and because of a calorie restriction due to decrease in carbohydrate content. However, the weight problems usually reappear after a crash or fad diet is stopped. The person often regains the lost weight after returning to one's normal diet that made him or her fat in the first place.

Formula Diets: Formula diets are supplied by pharmaceutical, dairy and food companies are in liquid, powder or solid form. The recommended daily quantities supply approximately 900 Calories and consists of 20 percent protein, 30 percent fat and 50 percent carbohydrate. The use of formula diets is simple, since they require no meal planning. However, one becomes sick of using formula diets as a substitute for regular tasty and varied meals. Therefore, formula diets are generally not carried as a long-term procedure. These are often discarded after a certain time and the person mostly returns to previous dietary habits and regains the weight lost. Formula diets may be of some value to those who occasionally need to lose a few pounds. On a long-term basis, they may be useful as a substitute for one meal a day.

Fasting or Starvation: Fasting is a severe treatment for obesity, with quick results that may or may not be lasting. Loss of 4 to 8 pounds a day during the first day or two is not rare, but most of this is due to water and sodium salt loss.

Vitamin supplements, black coffee and tea and sometimes low-calorie foods such as celery, are included as a part of the diet schedule. The usual great difficulty is that one regains the weight, once he is off the diet, so that all the sufferings of hunger end up in vain. Starvation treatment can also lead to serious complications, particularly in individuals with a history of gout or cardiac, renal, cerebral or hepatic disorders, and should be tried only in desperate situation under medical supervision.

Other treatments for extreme cases of obesity, which are practiced by medical professionals are, surgey (Jejunoileal Bypass, Gastric Bypass), hormonal therapy and jaw wiring. The techniques such as laxatives, diuretics, and liquid protein diets are dangerous means of reducing body fat, and should be avoided. The compulsive dieters with a condition of anorexia nervosa often try bizarre practices such as vomiting. Obviously, vomiting is never recommended as a method of weight control.

Behavior Modification: This is one of the recent diet techniques. An alternate acceptable behavior can be used to replace a particular set of environmental situations associated with eating. The overweight person gains insight into the factors that influence his or her eating behavior and learns methods for controlling the factors or the eating response to them, so that the end result is new eating and activity habits, weight loss and sustained maintenance of the lower weight.

Some of the common eating behavior modifications which are often suggested are as follows:
1. Replace the habit of eating snacks while watching television with sewing, painting or writing a letter.
2. In the kitchen, put something in your mouth such as chewing gum or a toothpick so that you cannot put food in your mouth.
3. Change the habit of eating candy while driving to singing with a radio.
4. If you feel hungry at a particular time, go for a walk at that time. Do the same during, a time of frustration—take a walk rather than eating.
5. Eat food only in one place, probably at the kitchen table, to control the frequency of eating. Also, eat only when hungry.
6. To control the rate of eating, chew for a long time and wait between each bite.
7. To control the amount of food eaten, serve meals on a smaller plate so that it appears as if there is more on it, or write down the amount of everything eaten, or eat half of enverything.

Similarly physical activity behavior may be modified. For example:
1. When driving to work, park half a mile away from work; whenever you travel a short distance, walk instead of taking a cab or a bus.
2. Whenever possible, use the stairs instead of elevators.
3. Replace cocktail hour or coffee breaks with exercise actitity.
4. Help yourself with gardening, mowing the lawn, washing the car, or shoveling the snow instead of hiring a help.

5. Play golf without a golf cart.
6. Replace power tools and appliances such as lawn care equipment, garage doors with manually operated devices.

These are only some of the examples of behavior modification, which can be kept in mind. Much of this comes from self-observation in the form of daily records, combined with will-power and efforts to change small details in one's life style as an investment in long-term weight control.

The Calorie-restricted Diet Plan: Calorie restriction is a popular and relatively straightforward method of weight reduction. The number of calories is decreased to the point where excess calories are no longer deposited as fat in the tissues, and the body is forced to draw on some of its own fat stores to meet energy needs. When this stage is reached, the individual will loose weight. A pound of body fat is equal to 3,500 Calories. Thus to lose one pound a week, one should consume fewer calories each day than expended (the reverse procedure should be followed to gain weight). Figure it this way . . . .

150 pounds desired weight
×15 Calories per pound for moderate activity/day
=2,250 Calories needed to maintain desired weight
−500 Calories daily deficit to lose one pound per week (i.e. total of 3,500 Calories in whole week)
=1,750 maximum daily Calories to be eaten to lose one pound per week.

If two pounds each week are to be lost, the calculation will simply include 1,000 Calories daily deficit leaving 1,250 maximum daily Calories to be eaten to lose two pounds per week. To try to lose more than two pounds per week is usually unwise because a rapid weight loss may leave a person tired, grumpy, and vulnerable to illness. Moreover, diets that promise quick loss are illusory. Their claims for loss of 4 to 8 pounds a day during the first day or two is true, but is mostly a water, not a fat. When you think about it, the loss of 4 or 8 pounds of fat in 1, 2 or even 4 days is impossible. A pound of body fat represents 3,500 Calories, and if you are moderately active 150-pounder—you need only 2,250 Calories per day. Even if you ate nothing and maintained regular activity, you can't lose even one pound, not to speak of 4 or 8 pounds. So if you want to lose fat, which is all you should want to lose, the loss must be gradual.

Obviously, low-calorie foods have an advantage in losing weight, because the total number of calorie-intake is less than high-calorie richer foods (see Table 4.9). For example, a cup of green beans contains 27 Calories, whereas a malted shake contains 502 Calories. The advantages of a low-calorie natural diet in weight control are discussed later in Chapter 5.

Physical Activity and Weight Control: Exercise in any form uses energy and will, therefore, burn calories. Table 4.10 lists various activities and calories required for each of them, as well as calculations of calories expended for the day. These table values are average values, applicable under average conditions when applied

Table 4.9 Energy equivalents of food calories expressed in minutes of activity.

Food	Calories	Walking (min)	Riding Bicycle (min)	Swimming (min)	Running (min)	Reclining (min)
Apple, Large	101	19	12	9	5	78
Bacon, 2 strips	96	18	12	9	5	74
Banana, small	88	17	11	8	4	68
Beans, green, 1 cup	27	5	3	2	1	21
Beer, 1 glass	114	22	14	10	6	88
Bread and butter	78	15	10	7	4	60
Cake, 1/12, 2-layer	356	68	43	32	18	274
Carbonated beverage, 1 glass	106	20	13	9	5	82
Carrot, raw	42	8	5	4	2	32
Cereal, dry, $\frac{1}{2}$cup, with milk and sugar	200	38	24	18	10	154
Cheese, cottage, 1 tbsp.	27	5	3	2	1	21
Cheese, Cheddar, 1 oz.	111	21	14	10	6	85
Chicken, fried, $\frac{1}{2}$ breast	232	45	28	21	12	178
Chicken, TV dinner	542	104	66	48	28	417
Cookie, plain, 148/lb	15	3	2	1	1	12
Cookie, chocolate chip	51	10	6	5	3	39
Doughnut	151	29	18	13	8	116
Egg, fried	110	21	13	10	6	85
Egg, boiled	77	15	9	7	4	59
French dressing, 1 tbsp.	59	11	7	5	3	45
Halibut steak, $\frac{1}{4}$ lb	205	39	25	18	11	158
Ham, 2 slices	167	32	20	15	9	128
Ice cream, 1/6 qt	193	37	24	17	10	148
Ice cream soda	255	49	31	23	13	196
Ice milk, 1/6 qt	144	28	18	13	7	111
Gelatin, with cream	117	23	14	10	6	90
Malted milk shake	502	97	61	45	26	386
Mayonnaise, 1 tbsp.	92	18	11	8	5	71
Milk, 1 glass	166	32	20	15	9	128
Milk, skim, 1 glass	81	16	10	7	4	62
Milk shake	421	81	51	38	22	324
Orange, medium	68	13	8	6	4	52
Orange juice, 1 glass	120	23	15	11	6	92
Pancake with syrup	124	24	15	11	6	95
Peach, medium	46	9	6	4	2	35
Peas, green, $\frac{1}{2}$ cup	56	11	7	5	3	43
Pie, apple, 1/6	377	73	46	34	19	290
Pie, raisin, 1/6	437	84	53	39	23	336
Pizza, cheese, 1/8	180	35	22	16	9	138
Pork chop, loin	314	60	38	28	16	242
Potato chips, 1 serving	108	21	13	10	6	83

Table 4.9 continued

Food	Calories	Activity				
		Walk-ing (min)	Riding Bicycle (min)	Swim-ming (min)	Run-ning (min)	Reclin-ing (min)
Sandwiches						
Club	590	113	72	53	30	454
Hamburger	350	67	43	31	18	269
Roast beef with gravy	430	83	52	38	22	331
Tuna fish salad	278	53	34	25	14	214
Sherbet, 1/6 qt	177	34	22	16	9	136
Shrimp, french-fried	180	35	22	16	9	138
Spaghetti, 1 serving	396	76	48	35	20	305
Steak, T-bone	235	45	29	21	12	181
Strawberry shortcake	400	77	49	36	21	308

SOURCE: Konishi, F.: *Food and Energy Equivalents of Various Activities.* J. Am. Diet. Assoc., 46: 187, 1965.

Table 4.10   A typical female college student's activities for one day.

Activity	Hours spent in activity	Calories per pound per hour	Total Calories per pound (Calories × Hours)
Asleep	8	0.4	3.2
Lying still, awake	1	0.5	0.5
Dressing and undressing	1	0.9	0.9
Sitting in class, eating, studying, talking	8	0.7	5.6
Walking	1	1.5	1.5
Standing	1	0.8	0.8
Driving a car	1	1.0	1.0
Running	$\frac{1}{2}$	4.0	2.0
Playing ping-pong	$\frac{1}{2}$	2.7	1.3
Writing	2	0.7	1.4
Total	24		18.2

Total Calories used per pound	18.2
Weight in pounds	× 115.0
Total Calories expended for the day	=2,093

SOURCE: Adapted from Helen S. Michell *et al.*, *Cooper's Nutrition in Health and Disease*, 15th ed, (Philadelphia 1968), pp. 50–51.

to an average person of a given body weight. Although these values are not precisely accurate for a particular individual, they do provide a good approximation of energy expenditure and are quite useful in establishing the appropriate caloric cost of an exercise program. As compared to dietary control, the exercise approach to weight reduction is less efficient. The amount of energy expended during physical activity is so low that a dieter would have to spend an inordinate amount of time exercising before achieving a substantial caloric deficit. However, regular exercise in addition to burning off extra calories helps to regulate the appetite, so that one is less likely to consume more calories than the body needs.

Underweight

Being underweight is a problem which is considerably less common than weighing too much. However, it should be paid proper attention. In underweight individuals, the resistance to disease is lowered, growth during childhood and adolescence is retarded, and efficiency for work or other activities is impaired. Underweight may be caused by (1) insufficient caloric intake of food to meet the needs of the person's activity, (2) poor absorption and utilization of the food consumed, (3) some kind of wasting disease such as tuberculosis, (4) psychological or emotional stress or psychological abnormality (Anorexia nervosa). Underweight problems such as faulty absorption of food may require medical treatment, but most often the cause of underweight is—simply—an inadequate food intake. Caloric treatment for the condition is the opposite of the treatment for overweight. The achievement of a positive caloric balance comes first; more calories have to be consumed each day than are expended.

To achieve a positive caloric balance, an allowance of 200 to 500 additional Calories should be planned. First of all determine the calories needed to meet the total energy requirement of the body on the basis of present weight. If a person normally needs 2,300 Calories to maintain present weight, his dietary needs would be 2,500 to 2,800 Calories to gain weight. The intake should be gradually increased to avoid gastric discomfort and periods of discouragement. The individual preferences to receive the additional calories may vary from extra portions of the usual foods served at meals, to between-meal nourishment, to more concentrated foods. The secret of a successful weight gaining program is to individualize extra calorie intake for each person and to include foods which the person really enjoys.

Concentrated calorie foods such as butter, margarine, cream, malted milk, eggnogs, and high-calorie desserts are especially useful to add calories. Moderate amounts of fat increase the palatability of the diet and increase the caloric value without dulling the appetite. Carbohydrate foods are the best ones to emphasize in adding calories, although all the basic foods should be represented in the daily food intake, with special emphasis on protein, minerals and vitamins. The B vitamins are especially good because they act as a possible appetite stimulant. Anyone trying to gain weight should remain or become reasonably active physically. Adding a pound or two a month is an achievable goal until the desired weight is reached. When this happens, there will have to be some adjustments in eating and exercise patterns so that a state of caloric balance is achieved.

Chapter **5**

The Natural Diet

The consumption of excessive meat and processed foods leads to an unbalanced diet, since they contain a great excess of protein, yet are almost completely lacking in carbohydrate, fiber, calcium, and health-promoting vitamins, originally derived from the plant kindgdom. However, these missing ingredients, essential part of good nutrition, can be provided by fresh vegetables, fruits, grains, and dairy products. A natural vegetarian diet, in fact, can supply all of the nutrition necessary for the human body. Perhaps it is not surprising that vegetarians have enjoyed good health for centuries. There are several examples of long-lived people—the Hunzans of Pakistan, the Abkhasians of the Soviet Union, and the Vilcabambams of Ecuador—whose diets contain little animal foods. While many factors, including high levels of exercise and low levels of stress, undoubtedly contribute to the longevity of these people, their natural vegetarian diet is likely to be a very significant factor. The "secret" of their natural diet is now supported by medical and scientific world that has recently realized, for example, the importance of carbohydrates and fiber, and the need for moderation in protein consumption to maintain a good health. Further support for a low-protein consumption is provided by a study on rats which has shown that a high-protein diet later in life shortened their life span (Ross and Bras, 1975, *Science*, Volume 190, p. 165).

What Is a Natural Diet?

Natural diet refers primarily to wholesome foods which resemble closely the original natural state in which they grow. They are not processed or preserved with chemicals and would include, for example, brown rice, not white; whole wheat, not refined flour; fresh, not canned vegetables; fruits, not fruit juices. Eaten raw or cooked, these foods are low in fats, cholesterol, protein, and highly refined carbohydrates such as sugars. They are high in mostly unrefined carbohydrates such as starches. These foods are not only safe and healthy, but are ideal for maintaining a proper weight level—without any restrictions on food quantity.

Many Americans are used to convenience-foods which may make the first step towards eating natural foods seem difficult. However, once that step is taken, and the food is tried and the rewards are understood, then the chances of adopting a natural diet are good. The process can be a gradual one, with adoption of various ingredients of the natural diet taking place at whatever pace is comfortable.

Natural foods are actually better suited to our bodies than are foods made popular by recent trends in eating. Natural foods are the basic foods which were available while our physiology evolved to its present complexity; these foods are in harmony with our digestive and metabolic machinery evolved over thousands of years.

A natural diet of wholesome foods primarily of plant origin comes close to being a vegetarian diet; except that dairy products are included in a natural diet. In fact, it will be appropriate to define here some of the terms for vegetarianism which the reader will come across in this chapter or elsewhere. The vegetarians who eat fruits, vegetables and dairy products are called *lactovegetarians*. The other terms used for vegetarians are *lacto-ovo-vegetarians* (those who eat eggs in addition to lactovegetarian foods) and *vegans* (those who eat fruits and vegetables only). The natural diet is probably close to that of lactovegetarians if they consume wholesome, unprocessed, unpreserved foods.

Why Adopt a Natural Vegetarian Diet?

Vegetarian foods provide an effective method of reducing the dangers of an over-rich diet; nutritionally you have nothing to lose. Recognition of vegetarianism as a part of health and longevity is now spreading. The number of voluntary vegetarians in Europe and the USA is estimated at several million. Some are motivated by aesthetic or moral ideas; they deplore the killing of animals and some of the methods of raising them for food. Many become vegetarians for hygienic reasons, spurning meat as a cause of digestive problems and disease, and a source of unhealthy chemicals and infectious organisms. Others simply believe that a vegetarian diet is more healthy. The unprocessed vegetarian foods are low in fat and cholesterol but are high in strarchy carbohydrates and fiber, and natural vitamins and minerals. The vegetable proteins can be as satisfying as meat protein. Proper combinations of vegetarian foods for good quality protein are explained later in this chapter.

For centuries the hardiest, most long-lived people in the world have thrived on these foods. President Thomas Jefferson, who lived to be eighty-three, believed his longevity was due to his vegetarian menus. He wrote, "I have lived temperately, eating little animal food, and not as an aliment, so much as a condiment for the vegetables which constitute my principal diet." Among other famous vegetarians were George Bernard Shaw, Leonardo da Vinci, Ralph Waldo Emerson, Henry David Thoreau, Benjamin Franklin, Mahatma Gandhi, Albert Schweitzer, and Gloria Swanson.

Vegetarian foods are not only healthy but are economical, so that even the poorest can afford them. Meat, on the other hand, is an expensive and inefficient nutrient. It is more efficient to use land for growing food for humans directly than for feeding animals which then are used as a food. Table 5.1 shows how many people, for the same period, could be supported by 10 acres of land in terms of vegetarian proteins compared with meat proteins. A 1,000 lb steer eats 5,250 lb of plant food in its lifetime. Its carcass weighs only 560 lb and from this the consumer will be able to buy only 280 lb in prime cuts of its meat—quite a significant reduction in the amount of available food.

Table 5.1   The economics of vegetarianism. The number of people fed by 10 acres of land in terms of vegetarian proteins compared with meat proteins.

Source of protein	No. of people fed
Soybean	61
Wheat	24
Corn	10
Meat	2

In view of the world-wide population explosion, our protein must come more and more from non-meat sources. The populated countries such as China and India for centuries have used more vegetable protein than animal protein. Less populated countries are now beginning to face the same problem. In the future vegetable protein foods, such as soybean products, are likely to become more important in our diet because they are cheaper to produce than animal protein (see Table 5.1). The ever increasing demand for protein can never be solved through meat—the world's resources are too limited to squander on the uneconomical conversion of plant to animal to human protein. Increasingly, people all over the world will have to rely on vegetable protein. If we all increase the use of vegetable proteins, food would be cheaper and more abundant.

Even if we are not concerned about the world food problem, dealing every day with the steadily rising cost of food, especially of meat and fish, is a good enough reason to learn about the utilization of plant proteins. Table 5.2 shows the relative cost of 54 grams of protein—the daily amount needed by a 150 pound adult—from

Table 5.2   The relative cost of 54 grams of protein from plant and animal sources. The daily recommended dietary allowance of protein for 150-pound adult.

Food	Amount	Cost (January 1980)
Dried beans, cooked	3 4/10 cups	$0.38
Peanut butter	13 1/2 tablespoons	0.54
Eggs	11 large	0.62
Chicken, whole	7/10 small broiler	0.73
Tuna, canned	7 1/2 ounces	1.08
Frankfurters	8 medium	1.65
Sardines, canned	10 ounces	1.73
Bacon, sliced	21 1/2 ounces	1.92
Bologna	16 ounces	2.16
Beef sirloin, with bone	12 ounces	2.21
Veal cutlets	9 1/2 ounces	2.81
Porterhouse steak, with bone	15 ounces	3.16
Lamb chops, loin	13 1/2 ounces	3.48

SOURCE: U. S. Department of Agriculture and Labor.

different foods. These figures are based on January 1980 prices by the U.S. Department of Agriculture and Labor. These will vary from time to time but should give a sense of the relative cost of our protein needs. Ounce for ounce, the protein in bologna costs four times as much as the protein in peanut butter. The protein in bacon is about five times, in beef about seven times and in lamb chops about 9 times as expensive as the same amount of protein from kidney beans.

Vegetarian foods provide an additional advantage of "eating low on the food chain." The higher on the food chain you eat, the greater your chances of accumulating large amounts of toxic materials present in tiny amounts in foods at the bottom of the chain. The meat protein, in fact, is called second-hand protein because the animal eats the vegetation, a primary source of protein, to build up its own protein which is then utilized by the meat eaters who eat that animal. The carnivorous animal protein is thus third hand and is often toxic to consume, and this is the reason that the meat people eat usually comes from vegetarian animals. Although fish appears to be an exception, health conscious people prefer small fish such as sardines, which are lower on the food chain, to bigger fish such as tuna. The reason is that big fish eat smaller fish, smaller fish eat still smaller fish, each with some pollutants or other toxins stored in its body, and therefore small fish at the lower end of the food chain are less likely to contain any pollutants or other toxic substances. This is, in fact, what has happened to birds of prey like falcons, ospreys, and eagles who eat big fish. These birds at the top of the food chain end up taking in such a large amount of pesticides such as DDT that their reproductive ability is severely damaged. The advantages of eating at the lower end of food chains has been substantiated by the data (1964–70) published in *Pesticides Monitoring Journal;* the plant foods at the lower end of food chains contain less pesticide residues than foods of animal origin. The vegetarians go right to the beginning of the food chain and from nuts, seed, beans, grains, and vegetables, they get protein first-hand from nature.

One could cite numerous other reasons for eating vegetarian foods, but the one we would realize in this chapter is simply that vegetarian food is good for you to enjoy the best of health. I would quote the common responses of many vegetarian people that refer to their personal experience rather than any nutritional aspects: (1) although the main quality for being a vegetarian is not eating meat, vegetarianism is more like an entire relationship with the world—a sensitive vibration; it is a spiritual position that we have arrived at—as our place here on earth, (2) there is something violent about meat-eating; you are constantly slaughtering animals for your gastronomic pleasure, (3) there is something nice and clean about eating grains; they are good for your body, (4) meat-eaters tend to "break" because they are not as adaptable; meat-eating leaves one feeling very heavy and sluggish; it also makes people more aggressive, (5) vegetarians have high levels of endurance and can work for longer hours.

What Does Biological and Evolutionary Evidence Tell Us About Being Vegetarians or Meat Eaters?

Although human beings are considered as omnivores who can eat both plant- and animal-food, our anatomical equipment leans heavily towards a vegetarian diet.

Our teeth are evolved to deal with tubers and seeds, not flesh. Our front teeth are large and sharp, good for biting; our canines are small—almost vestigial compared to a tiger's; our molars are flattened; and our jaws are mobile for grinding food into the small bits we are able to swallow. In contrast, carnivores have long, strong, pointed canine teeth; their upper premolars and lower molars are also large and better designed for cutting than grinding—these slice through flesh like a pair of shears; their jaw moves very little from side to side, limiting their ability to grind food. Dr. Alan Walker of Johns Hopkins University conducted microscopic analyses of the wear patterns on the teeth of our humanlike ancestors, which indicate that we have evolved from fruit eaters, not flesh eaters. The fossil teeth of these early hominids contain none of the scratch marks found on the teeth of animals that gnaw on bones and flesh.

As for the digestive tract, here, too, we are more like the herbivores. Carnivores have a comparatively short, smooth intestinal tract, only about three times the length of their body. Since they eat raw meat that decomposes rapidly, they must digest it fast and get rid of the wastes before toxins accumulate. The human intestines are long—twelve times as long as the torso—and highly convoluted, allowing us to digest substances that take a long time to be broken down and absorbed. Plant foods, with their large amounts of fiber, are just such substances. But whether plant or animal, food takes its time passing through the human digestive system. This leaves animal waste in the body for far longer than it remains in carnivores, and as discussed later, this fact may be related to the high rates of cancer of the colon and rectum among people who eat a lot of meat.

Early humans required meat at times for survival, but analyses of fossilized human fecal matter shows that they subsisted mainly on vegetation—fruits, nuts, tubers, berries, and grains. The invention of agriculture—the cultivation of crops for food—further assured a steady supply of edible plants for our acncestors. But it was a long time before animals were domesticated and raised for food, and even then, they were infrequently consumed. More likely they served as suppliers of such renewable foods as milk and eggs. In conclusion, we are biologically constructed as vegetarians, not as consumers of vast quantities of meat.

Nutritional Consideration of a Natural Vegetarian Diet

The overemphasis on high-protein consumption by meat-oriented food writers of the Western world has undoubtedly contributed to some of the skepticism about the safety of a vegetarian diet. Vegetarians in Europe and America are like left-handed people in a right-handed world. Almost all vegetarians and those thinking of becoming one, are most concerned about getting an adequate supply of protein.

If you are on a reasonably well-balanced diet, you need have no fear of getting inadequate protein. A vegetarian diet can be nutritionally sound for all age groups, differing from a normal diet only in the sort of foods supplying the essential nutrients. Although the body must get sufficient supply of these life-sustaining chemicals, their source—whether from meat or non-meat foods—does not matter at all.

The statistical data on athletic records have indicated that players on vegetarian diets performed as well or even better than those on high-meat diets. Back in 1904, vegetarian and non-vegetarian students were compared as to how many times they could squeeze a grip meter in quick, succession. The vegetarians scored an average of 69 times; the non-vegetarians averaged 38. More recently, nine Swedish athletes tested for endurance on a stationary bicycle lasted nearly three times longer after a three-day diet high in vegetables and grains but low in protein than they did after three days of a high-meat diet. If you are still not convinced, note the achievements of vegetarian athletes recounted by Vic Sussman in his book, *A Vegetarian Alternative*. Paavo Nurmi, a Finn, trained on a vegetarian diet, set twenty world running records between 1920 and 1932. Bill Pickering, a British vegetarian, swam the English Channel in 1956 in record-breaking time. Murray Rose, an Australian who had been a vegetarian since the age of 2, at age 17 became the youngest Olympic triple gold medal winner for swimming events in 1956.

Since the quality of mixed cereal and legume proteins matches that of meat and fish proteins, vegetarian diets have protein values similar to those of mixed diets, provided proper combination of foods and adequate quantities are consumed. For example, if you depend entirely on white rice for your protein, you would most likely become protein deficient because rice provides less than 5 percent of usable or complete protein (grams of protein per 100 Calories adjusted by quality score or net protein utilization and then expressed in terms of protein Calories per 100 total Calories), which is the minimum safe level recommended for adults by the World Health Organization. The protein value of beans is about 20 percent usable protein. The combination of rice and beans, however, raises the usable protein value up to 50 percent. This happens because the amino acids in the two foods complement each other. The rice is low in lysine but has a surplus of the sulfur-containing amino acids (e.g. cystine), while the beans are low in the sulfur containing amino acids but have a surplus of lysine. Similarly, eating wheat and beans together can increase the protein actually usable by the body by about 33 percent.

Table 5.3 shows the amino acid strengths and weaknesses of various food groups; and Table 5.4 lists the typical combinations of these various food groups to make dishes with complete protein. As a rule of thumb, keep three simple combinations in mind: (1) combine legumes with grains; (2) combine legumes with nuts and seeds; (3) combine eggs or dairy products with any vegetable protein.

Buddhist monks in Korea who eat an extremely large amount of white rice—60 percent of their calories—enjoy good health because they supplement their rice with beans and other nutritious foods. Many vegetarians in poorer countries are able to survive in good health with no animal food because they get quality

Table 5.3 Amino acid strengths and weaknesses of various food groups.

Food group	Weaknesses	Strengths
Legumes	Tryptophan, Methionine, Cystine*	Lysine, Isoleucine
Grains	Lysine, Isoleucine	Tryptophan, Methionine, Cystine*
Seeds and Nuts	Lysine, Isoleucine (except cashews and pumpkin seeds)	Tryptophan, Methionine, Cystine*
Other Vegetables	Isoleucine, Methionine, Cystine*	Tryptophan, Lysine
Eggs	None	Tryptophan, Lysine, Methionine, Cystine*
Milk Products	None	Lysine

Note: To achieve balanced protein, combine food groups as given in the next table (Table 5.4) so that the amino acid strengths of one compensate for the weaknesses of the other.

*Although cystine is not an essential amino acid, its presence in foods spares methionine, which is essential.

protein from combinations of rice and beans or wheat and beans (malnourished vegetarians in poorer countries, however, are due to lack of sufficient food availability). Some food writers such as Frances Lappé (author of a best-seller, *Diet for a Small Planet*, Ballantine Books, New York) suggest beans and rice in the balanced proportion of 1 to 2.7 in order to maximize protein values; however, such precision is not necessary, and vegetarians have enjoyed good health by combining grains and beans to their individual taste for thousands of years.

In most traditional cultures, grains and beans are eaten together in a variety of food combinations. In Mexico, corn tacos and *tortillas* are eaten with pinto beans. The peasants of Cuba eat rice with black beans. In India, *Chapati* (flat unleavened whole wheat bread) are eaten with *dal* (mung bean, lentils, peas and various other legumes). In China and Japan, *tofu* (bean curd) is eaten together with rice. Among other combinations that provide good protein values are cereals (grains) and milk, macaroni and cheese, grains and egg (for lacto-ovo-vegetarians), beans and nuts or seeds, and brewer's yeast and grains. To exploit this complementary effect, you can make dishes and plan meals with the help of Table 5.3 and 5.4 so that the protein in one food fills the amino acid deficiencies in another food.

As for amounts of protein, three things are worth bearing in mind. First, most meat eaters are already consuming twice as much protein as they really need. Second, the protein in milk and eggs is more efficiently used by the body than that in meat, fish, or poultry, so relatively little goes a long way nutritionally. Third, legumes—especially soybeans—contain the largest precentage of protein among vegetable foods and are in the same ball park as many meats. If legumes play a central role in your diet, you're not likely to shortchange yourself on protein.

Table 5.4 Typical vegetarian dishes with complete protein.

Grains with Legumes

Rice with lentils	Macaroni enriched with soy flour
Rice with black-eyed peas	Bean soup with toast
Peanut-butter sandwich	Falafel (chickpea pancake) with pita bread
Bean taco	

Grains with Milk

Oatmeal with milk	Macaroni and cheese
Wheat flakes with milk	Cheese sandwich
Rice pudding	Creamed soup with noodles or rice
Pancakes and waffles	Quiche
Bread and muffins made with milk	Meatless lasagna
Pizza	Granola with milk

Legumes with Seeds

Bean curd with sesame seeds	Bean soup with sesame meal
Hummus (chickpea and sesame paste)	

Grains with Eggs

Rice pudding	Egg-salad sandwich
Kasha (buchwheat groats)	Noodle pudding
Fried rice	French toast
Oatmeal cookies	
Quiche	

Other Vegetables with Milk or Eggs

Potato salad	Cheese and potato soup
Mashed potatoes with milk	Vegetable omelet
Eggplant Parmesan	Escalloped potatoes
Broccoli with cheese sauce	Spinach salad with sliced egg
Cream of pumpkin soup	

Thus, one cup of cooked soybeans contains about 20 grams of protein—as much protein as three Frankfurters, or 1/4-pound hamburger, or 18 ounces of milk, or 3 ounces of cheese! Each would supply two-thirds of a 60-pound child's daily protein needs, nearly half the recommended protein allowance for a 120-pound adult, and a third the amount needed by a 170-pound man.

If you are doubtful about adequate consumption of protein, its deficiency can be observed from your body's condition. Because nails, hair, and skin require newly synthesized protein for growth and health, their condition is usually a good indication of whether or not you are getting enough protein. Similarly, notice whether or not abrasions heal quickly. If they don't, you may be seriously lacking protein in your diet. A natural diet, followed with understanding of nutritional needs, however, would never lead to this problem.

There is certainly a tendency for vegetarians to have a lower calorie intake than people on mixed diets. This is largely because, in the absence of meat-eating, vegetarians' fat intake is lower—an advantage in view of the association of high fat consumption with heart disease. However, if higher intake of calories or fat is

Table 5.5 Comparative amounts of nutrients in various foods.

| Food Source | Percent of | | | | | | Calories per 100g (3.5 ounces) |
	Protein	Carbohy-drates	Fat	Vitamins and minerals	Fiber	Water	
Cereal grain							
Wheat	13.50	70.00	3.00	2.00	1.50	10.00	330
Rice	7.00	76.50	1.00	2.00	1.50	12.00	360
Rye	7.50	72.00	2.00	2.00	1.50	15.00	330
Oats	11.50	66.00	9.00	2.00	1.50	10.00	400
Corn and Millet	11.00	69.00	4.50	2.00	1.50	12.00	350
Barley	8.00	75.00	1.50	2.00	1.50	12.00	350
Nuts and Legumes							
Nuts-almonds	16.00	16.00	59.00	2.00	2.00	5.00	600
Kidney beans	24.00	55.00	2.00	2.50	4.50	12.00	330
Vegetables							
Brassicas-broccoli	3.50	5.00	0.25	0.25	1.00	90.00	35
Salad Leaves-lettuce	1.50	3.00	0.25	0.25	1.00	94.00	20
Root Vegetables-carrots	1.50	8.00	0.00	0.50	1.00	89.00	20
Tubers-potato	2.00	17.00	0.00	0.50	0.50	80.00	80
Stalk Vegetables-celery	2.25	3.00	0.25	0.50	1.00	93.00	15
Fruit Vegetables-tomato	0.50	3.00	0.00	0.50	1.00	95.00	15
Bulb Vegetables-onion	1.50	7.00	0.00	0.50	1.00	90.00	30
Mushrooms	2.00	0.00	0.25	0.25	5.50	92.00	10
Fruit							
Apples-Pears	0.50	13.00	0.25	0.25	2.00	84.00	60
Prunus Fruit-plums	1.00	13.00	0.25	0.25	0.50	85.00	50
Citrus Fruit-orange	0.75	10.00	0.25	0.50	0.50	80.00	40
Grapes	0.75	17.25	0.25	0.25	0.50	81.00	75
Banana	0.75	18.00	0.25	0.25	0.75	80.00	80
Berries-strawberries	1.00	8.00	0.75	0.25	3.00	87.00	40
Dried Fruit-raisins	3.00	68.00	1.00	2.00	3.00	23.00	300
Milk							
Cow's milk	3.00	4.50	4.00	1.00	0.00	87.00	65
Cheese-Cheddar	25.00	2.00	29.00	4.00	0.00	40.00	400

required, cereal grains contain more than 65 percent carbohydrates and nuts are more than 50 percent fat (see Table 5.5).

The vegetarian diet, with its protein-rich cereals and legumes, is certainly an excellent source of natural vitamins and minerals that people need, and vegetarians tend to have relatively high intakes of calcium, vitamin B, and vitamin C. However, vegetarians living exclusively on vegetables (vegans) have a low dietary intake of two vitamins, B_{12} and D. For these people, B_{12} tablets can provide extra vitamin B_{12} if needed, although for most people on a natural diet, fresh milk and cheese can supplement the diet. Moreover, vitamin B_{12} supply is not needed regularly since it is stored in the liver; the storage supply can last for about 5 years. A deficiency of vitamin B_{12} can cause anemia and in extreme cases nervous disorders. Vitamin D is important for the bone development of children, but adults do not generally need vitamin D in their diet. Since it is synthesized under the skin in the presence of sunlight, and if one gets enough sunlight vitamin D deficiency is unlikely. In fact, supplemented milk and margarines supply more than adequate amounts of vitamin D and it has been recommended that fortification of foods other than milk and margarine be reduced or discontinued for the U.S. population.

To assure proper growth and development, infants and young children should include animal protein as milk and milk products or eggs. Although a few vegan communities are raising infants according to carefully spelled out vegan nutritional guidelines, in general, this is unadvisable.

How Healthy Is It To Be a Meateater?

To many old civilizations it seemed uncivilized to kill animals. This is what Thoreau had in mind when he wrote in *Walden:* "I have no doubt that it is a part of the destiny of the human race, in its gradual improvement, to leave off eating animals, as surely as the savage tribes have left off eating each other when they came in contact with the more civilized." In the ancient Hindu sacred book *Bhagavad Gita* meat, alcohol, fish, eggs and hot spicy substances are classified as stimulating foods, whereas natural vegetarian foods are considered under the category of pure food. Pure food is believed to bring purity and calmness to the mind, and to be soothing and nourishing to the body. For these reasons, pure food is thought to be preferred by spiritually and mentally advanced people, while stimulating food, believed to arouse animal passion and a restless state of mind, would belong to average worldly people.

As quoted above, such philosophical and religious reasons against meat consumption may seem a thin basis for avoiding or reducing meat and adopting a vegetarian diet today; however, various unhealthy effects of a diet high in meat are being uncovered by recent scientific findings. A diet high in meat, for example, is suggested as a contributing factor in uric acid diseases. A pound of liver contains 19 grains of uric acid and a pound of beefsteak 14 grains, whereas the amount of uric acid the body produces and eliminates through the kidneys daily is only about 6 grains. As a person's liver and kidneys are not able to deal with the extra intake, the uneliminated uric acid becomes the seedbed of gout, rheumatism, headaches, epilepsy, convulsions, nervousness, etc. The statistical records indicate that the consumption of large quantities of meat is also a contributing factor to heart problems, and even cancer.

A comparative study of diet and heart disease in seven countries showed that the Finns, who consumed the most animal fats, also had the highest death rate. Americans were next, but the Greeks and Italians, who eat relatively little animal fat, were near the bottom of the heart-disease death-rate list. In Japan, where very little fat of any kind is eaten, the heart-disease death-rate is lower than in any other industrialized nation, despite high rates of high blood pressure and cigarette smoking. In America, Seventh-Day Adventists, most of whom eat no meat or poultry, have only 60 percent the amount of heart diseases as compared to other Americans. In Boston a study of 116 vegetarians showed that they had lower blood pressures and cholesterol levels than comparable groups of meat-eating young adults. But those vegetarians who consumed dairy products and eggs more than five times a week had higher blood pressures and cholesterol levels than those who ate these animal foods less often or not at all.

Even those vegetarians who eat dairy products and eggs, which contain saturated animal fat and cholesterol, are not likely to come anywhere near the fat and cholesterol content of the typical mixed American diet. Most people who can afford meat probably eat too much of it. Conventional American meals make excessive meat-eating almost inevitable; there is a substantial amount of fat in most of the meat and only a small proportion of it is polyunsaturated. Saturated fats (mostly from animal origin or hydrogenated fat) in human diets influence amounts of plasma lipids and serum cholesterol. Increased levels of both cholesterol and lipids result in hardening of arteries which cause such vascular disorders as hypertension or high blood pressure. By substituting saturated with highly unsaturated fats (e.g. from safflower, corn and cotton seed oil), amount of plasma lipid and serum cholesterol is lowered. The removal of both saturated as well as unsaturated fats from the diet is even more effective in lowering blood cholesterol. In fact, the influence of fat on increasing serum cholesterol is much more effective than direct dietary intake of cholesterol. Lowered consumption of fat, particularly the saturated fat of meat origin, therefore, can reduce considerably the risks of lipid and cholesterol related heart problems.

Research findings during the last decade have revealed that the same kind of diet high in animal fats and cholesterol that sets the stage for heart-disease may also contribute to the growth of cancers of the colon, breast, and uterus. For example, among the Seventh-Day Adventists, most of whom eat no meat or poultry, these cancers are quite rare, but they are leading cancers among other meat-eating Americans. There are several possible explanations for this relationship. With regard to colon cancer, diets rich in saturated fats and cholesterol may result in large accumulations of natural cancer-promoting chemicals in the gut. And the relatively low fiber content of such diets may result in slow-moving bowels and prolonged contact of the cancer-promoting chemicals with body tissues. As for cancers of the breast and uterus, their growth is stimulated by estrogen hormones. A diet high in fat and cholesterol results in the production of estrogen-like hormones in the gut, and similar hormones are produced in body fat.

The above findings, therefore, do support the suggestions that reduced or no consumption of meat can decrease the dangers of heart, cancer, and uric acid related problems and increase your chances of enjoying good health. The aim here is not to belittle the food value of meat but to emphasize that without it, you can not only have a nutritionally sound diet but also at the same time reduce the risks associated with higher meat consumption.

A Natural Diet Can Prevent Diseases

Natural diet can be used as a medicine chiefly in the preventive sense by eating food in its natural state as much as possible. It is believed that many ailments are caused by accumulation of poison through improper eating and that a steady intake of selected foods fortifies the body against various health problems. For example, sinus congestion is associated with an over-consumption of mucus- and acid-forming foods; replacing fruits and vegetables for milk and meat should relieve a congestion problem. Freshly made vegetable and fruit juices are very good for those who suffer from chronic ailments, yet raw vegetable juices should not be thought of as a drug to cure ailments. They are rather the most vital rebuilding and regenerating foods that the body can use for construction. If one intends to feed only on freshly made juice for a week or two, one can drink several pints of juice a day. At times one can feel discomfort from feeding on raw juices, usually because of the stirring up of poisons accumulated in the system, but soon energy and vigor return when the toxins are eliminated. Dr. John Harvey Kellogg (of the family that started the cereal company), Medical Director, Battle Creek (Michigan) Sanitarium, used fruits, cereals, and fresh vegetables to make an "antitoxic diet" for his patients.

Fasting is another way to get rid of toxins and poisonous matter, especially during sickness; in addition to giving rest to the digestive system, fasting forces the body to use accumulated fat where toxins are stored. The modern medicine-oriented man, rather than eliminating accumulated poisons, uses pain-killing drugs to suppress pain, and thus, merely adds more poison through the drugs themselves. Illnesses such as fever and headache are nature's way of warning us that our bodies are not functioning normally. Some health clinics in Europe go so far as to claim that fever, by raising temperature, actually works to the benefit of the body by activating antibodies that help fight invasion of germs. By using aspirin or other pain relieving drugs, we can dull the pain, and the warning signals, but the source of trouble is still there and eventually may result in greater disturbances.

As mentioned in the preceding section, cancers of the colon, breast, and uterus are quite rare among primarily vegetarian groups such as Seventh-Day Adventists in comparison to meat-eating Americans. In addition to other possible explanations for this relationship (see the preceding section on "How Healthy Is It To Be a Meateater"), a variety of vegetable foods and fruit, including Brussels sprouts, cauliflower, broccoli, turnips, cabbage, spinach, celery, citrus fruits, beans, and seeds, can stimulate the production of anticancer enzymes in the body. Dr. Saxon Graham, professor of social and preventive medicine at State University of New York, found that chemicals in vegetables belonging to the cabbage family block the action of certain cancer-causing substances. In view of these observations, the consumption of vegetables and fruits as mentioned above should reduce the chances of having cancer.

Among the other observed effects of a vegetarian diet is a greater bone density among older persons and a lower incidence of osteoporosis and its complications. The mechanism for this is unclear but one hypothesis is that avoidance of meat creates less of an acid residue to be buffered by calcium salts drawn from bone stores.

The natural diet, because of its high fiber content, has also been shown to be especially beneficial in helping to prevent certain heart and digestive system related diseases as discussed in the next section on fiber.

High-fiber Food in the Natural Diet and the Role of Fiber in Health

Wholesome natural food eaten raw provides an excellent source of roughage or fiber which is often lacking in a processed food and a meat. The importance of fiber in health has become so obvious that no longer can nutritionists avoid paying attention to its role.

Fiber is the cell wall material of plants which adds roughage or bulk to our food; and it is not digestible except for small amounts broken down by intestinal bacteria. Chemically it is made up of cellulose, hemicellulose, lignin, pectin and cutin. The quantity of each constituent depends on the specific plant and may vary within each species. The most common sources of fiber in our diets are whole grains, fruits, and vegetables.

Fiber has been shown to prevent common noninfective diseases of the colon, such as constipation, diverticulosis (a disease in which little pouches form along the intestinal tract but most frequently in the colon), and cancer. Fiber affects stool bulk, softness, and transit time. It has been theorized that a high-fiber diet by cutting bowel transit time, allows less time for bacteria in the colon to produce carcinogens (cancer-producing substances). Rural Ugandans who hardly ever get cancer of the colon, eat considerable fiber. Their average bowel transit time is 36 hours, compared to 77 hours for British men who consumed lower-fiber diets like most of the Americans. Although cancer of the colon has also been claimed to be related to fat consumption, this does not eliminate the possibility that fiber plays a role in the disease. A high-fiber diet may also protect against a variety of other diseases, including heart disease (by lowering blood cholesterol), appendicitis, gallstones, hemorrhoids, and diabetes.

The findings about the role of dietary fiber in lowering blood cholesterol are among the most encouraging for heart patients. The types of fiber which have beneficial effects are the ones consumed from natural foods, but not bran. Bran is more than 90 percent cellulose and has no beneficial effect on cholesterol levels. Pectins (found in most fruits), guar gum (found in beans), and the fiber in rolled oats and carrots are especially useful in lowering blood cholesterol. When patients were given 5 grams of guar gum before each meal, cholesterol dropped an average of 10.6 percent over and above the reduction caused by the drugs. Scottish researchers showed that eating 7 ounces of raw carrots at breakfast every day for three weeks could reduce cholesterol levels by 11 percent and increase the amount of fat excreted by 50 percent. Fiber's cholesterol-lowering effect may result from its ability to increase the excretion of bile acids, which are made from cholesterol. Physiologists at the University of Southampton in England showed that the fiber consumed by vegetarians can lower blood pressure. Its influence on blood-sugar level and insulin requirements is another beneficial effect of a dietary fiber. By including fiber in their diets, Dr. J. W. Anderson, V. A. Hospital, Lexington, Kentucky, found that some diabetics have been able to get along without insulin or other antidiabetic medication. Here, too, pectin and guar gum are the most effective plant fibers. Another popular plus for fiber is that it encourages weight loss (see next section).

As for how much fiber you should eat, no one can yet say. Vegetarians, however, should not be concerned. The studies have shown that on average vegetarians get over 50 percent more fiber than meat eaters. Non-vegetarians and those who consume excessive amounts of processed foods and refined grains are likely to have lower fiber consumption. They do not need to buy a jar of fiber pills or boxes of bran and pectin, all they need to do is to increase consumption of wholesome vegetarian foods. In fact, calculating the amount of fiber consumed is not necessary, but including whole grain foods, fresh fruits, and vegetables in the diet should be the main concern. Since fiber is relatively hard to digest and may also cause excessive intestinal gas problems, a steady increase of fiber from natural foods only, without the use of added fiber, is advisable; these problems, however, are temporary and subside in a few weeks when the bacterial population of your digestive system adapts to increased fiber intake.

Importance of a Natural Diet in Weight Control and Regularity

Obesity is rare in populations where a lot of natural fruits, vegetables and whole grains are consumed. But excess weight is a common problem in developed countries like the United States, where the progress of scientific and technical development has led to the common use of processed and refined foods which are concentrated in protein, minerals and vitamins. At least two effects of this move of getting away from natural fruits, vegetables, and whole grain foods are obvious. One is the high caloric intake resulting from the decreased volume of processed foods. In other words, overconsumption of calories to fill the stomach, which leads to an overweight problem. A second but related problem due to processed high protein foods is loss of roughage or bulk, which, as mentioned in the preceding section, results in irregularity and digestive system problems such as the intestinal diverticular disease. The ability of fibrous foods to counter the problem of constipation, in fact, has long been known to the medical profession and the general public. In the United States alone more than 700 different laxative preparations are sold over the counter, and one percent of all prescriptions are for laxatives. Many of these drugs act as stimulants to the colon, and their repeated use can lead to a chronic inability of the colon to act on its own. These drugs may also cause cramps, diarrhea, and excessive loss of fluids and essential minerals. The sensible way to treat constipation, therefore, is to consume wholesome natural foods, and not the use the laxative drugs. These and other problems related to low fiber intake became obvious only after getting away from natural foods.

The effectiveness of natural diet in weight control could be due to several reasons. In addition to giving the dieter a feeling of fullness in the stomach, which reduces the appetite, studies on high fiber diet claim that it requires more chewing. Chewing (mastication) diminishes the sensation of abnormal appetite that compels a person to eat more than is needed. This results in a diet that responds only to natural hunger. It is also possible that because of the decrease in bowel transit time caused by high fiber content of natural foods, small amounts of the fat and protein you eat are excreted. Therefore, a few of the calories you eat really don't count. A high fiber content may also inhibit absorption of nutrients through the intestine, thus encouraging weight loss. Although some of the nutrients not absorbed may be categorized as "essential," the consumption of protein and other nutrients by most Americans is so much in excess of what is needed that this degree of loss is not likely to be a problem.

Treating an Overweight Problem by Adopting a Natural Vegetarian Diet

The purpose of this chapter or of the whole book is not to convert anyone to vegetarianism but to bring to your attention the comparative food values of various meat and non-meat sources; and to emphasize strongly the benefits that can come from simply changing eating habits rather than going on crash diets or joining some similar tortuous weight loss program.

The various programs to treat overweight and the reasons for their failure are discussed in Chapter 4. Unfortunately, most of these weight loss programs are not really permanent solutions because sooner or later you are likely to discontinue the program and therefore face the same weight problem once again. Moreover, sudden weight loss (such as can be due to any of the weight loss programs) can be accompanied by side effects of mental stress or sickness which would require visits to a doctor either before starting a weight loss program or after the weight loss. On the other hand, if you follow nutritional advice and develop good eating habits, these habits are likely to last forever.

Considering the overweight problem and weight-consciousness of Americans, it is surprising that more people have not become vegetarians—perhaps lack of awareness about vegetarian nutrition and cooking has been a major contributing factor. Eating simple, low fat, low calorie food of plant origin will not only help you in losing weight but your body will feel light and energetic rather than sluggish. As you see in this natural diet chapter, vegetables are very low in calories and high in health-promoting natural minerals and vitamins; furthermore, their bulk fills the stomach and thus satisfies the appetite. For example, 5 ounces of meat provides 500 Calories, whereas the same amount of cooked kidney beans provide only 167 Calories. Green beans and other fresh vegetables are even lower in calories, and on the average provide less than one fourth of the calories than that of kidney beans. A lunch of vegetable soup, a slice of whole-grain bread, and a cottage cheese and fruit salad has a third fewer calories than the cheeseburger lunch (and far, far less saturated fat and cholesterol). And for the caloric value of a 6-ounce steak, a vegetarian could eat 3 cups of rice or a whole pound of noodles or, to be more reasonable, the vegetarian could eat a very generous serving of a casserole of noodles, vegetables, and cheese, which would eliminate the need for the potatoes and carrots in the steak dinner. A meal of a cup of brown rice and lentils, two slices of whole-grain bread (or a large baked potato) with margarine, ½ cup each of carrots and peas, a lettuce and tomato salad with dressing, and a fruit salad containing a banana, one apple, one orange, 2 tablespoons of raisins, and half a dozen walnuts, would contain about 890 Calories (610 less than the steak dinner) and leave the diner positively stuffed. While this is not typical of a meal that might be prepared by an experienced vegan, it does illustrate the huge amounts of food a vegan can consume without exceeding the body's caloric needs.

According to natural diet philosophy, it is not necessary to become a food crank and weigh, measure, and analyze every mouthful of food. It is simply true that you are unlikely to grow fat by including good amounts of fresh vegetables and fruits in your diet. Most of these are over 80 percent water and contain only the merest traces of fat and very little carbohydrate. The young vegetarians studied in Boston weighed an average 33 pound less than the meat-eating comparison group, because as mentioned earlier, a vegetarian diet is bulky and filling, and it's hard to eat more calories than your body burns. As a result, most people lose weight when they start a vegetarian diet. Those who are strict vegetarians (vegans) and eat no dairy products or eggs may actually have a hard time consuming enough calories to maintain their weight. Clearly, for an obese person a vegetarian diet with its naturally lower caloric content is a blessing. However, a normal (or underweight) person does need to make some adjustments in both total food intake and intake of adequate amounts of foods such as legumes, cereals and nuts to add calories for achieving an appropriate caloric balance.

To suit the wide range of tastes and dietary habits of Westerners, meat analogues may be included to replace meat until you start enjoying exclusively natural foods. Meat analogues are made with soybeans, molded into common meat foods such as sausages and burgers. You have probably seen them in the market as textured vegetable protein (TVP) which is a popular, inexpensive, and highly nourishing meat extender among non-vegetarians in many parts of the United States.

To make the ersatz "meat," first the oil is pressed out of the soybeans and then the carbohydrates are removed, leaving a honeylike slurry of pure protein. This is pumped through a "spinnerette"—a showerheadlike device with microscopic holes—and as the protein emerges from the holes, it hits an acid bath that converts it into fibers. After being neutralized and washed, the tasteless, odorless, off-white fibers are mixed with flavorings, colorings, fat, water, and sometimes egg white as a binder. By varying the stretch on the fibers as they go through the spinnerette, they can be spun into a variety of meatlike textures.

A second process for making vegetable meat analogues uses soybean flour or defatted soybean concentrate instead of isolated protein. This is mixed with water and flavorings, subjected to heat and pressure; and then forced through small holes of various sizes and shapes. The resulting product is then cooked and ready to eat. Or it may be frozen, canned, or dried. The spun protein can be sliced, cubed, cut into chunks, ground into bits or molded into rolls. In addition to soybeans, textured vegetable protein can be made from peanut, cottonseed, sunflower, safflower, and other oil seeds.

Because their nutritive content can be precisely controlled, meat analogues can be prepared with the identical food value of the foods they imitate. In fact, they may be healthier than the "real meat" because they can be made with little or no animal fats and cholesterol and sometimes fewer calories. The analogues are also easy to store and to prepare.

Some people who have become vegetarians because they want a "natural" diet object to the extensive processing and large numbers of additives and salt used in making meat analogues. But for others, the meat imitations make it esay to give up the foods they grew up on and instead stick to a vegetarian diet. Even if you are not a vegetarian, you may find some of the analogues to be attractive, economical, and healthy alternatives to meat. TVP can go a long way to stretch your food dollar (see Appendix E for a list of manufacturers of meat analogues and of stores that are likely to carry their products).

Even if you have no interest in vegetarianism, there's no reason why you should have animal protein at every meal or even every day. By including vegetarian dishes in your daily menu and adapting the vegetarian approach to menu planning, you can greatly reduce your dependence on animal protein and especially on high-fat, high-calorie meats.

Vegetarian Foods for Health

Vegetarianism is an alternative that can offer a surprisingly tasty and varied diet which can be nutritionally sound, and it saves money as well. With proper cooking the taste of vegetables can be more enjoyable than that of fat-saturated bacon and hot dogs. Choose vegetables and fruits of your choice and make them a major part of daily meals. Avoid the saturated fats and concentrated proteins of meat origin; satisfy your protein needs by selecting legumes such as soybeans along with cereals and milk for obtaining all the amino acids.

The importance given to meat in western diets is curious considering that the choice of meat is limited to beef, lamb, pork and chicken—only a minority of people venture beyond these. By comparison, plants can give an infinite variety of natural flavors to a diet, without the need of elaborate artifice by the cook. Provided a vegetarian knows about protein sources, there is a wide variety of vegetarian food that can replace the protein supplied in an ordinary diet by meat, fish and poultry.

Our thinking about the need for huge amounts of animal protein is changing as we are learning that an overabundance of animal protein actually can be detrimental to health. Without doubt, vegetables rank high among the good ingredients of a diet; what is required is a reasonably good knowledge about vegetarian foods. If you choose your foods properly, you will not have to take any vitamin or mineral supplements. Good nutrition is always balanced and complete, but we don't have to be biochemists or nutritionists to keep our diets balanced. The simple and easy way is to include each of these four groups of foods in the daily menu: (1) bread and cereal group (four servings), (2) protein group—nuts and legumes (two servings), (3) fruit-vegetable group (four servings), (4) milk group (two, three or four servings for adults, children and teens, respectively).

Bread and Cereal Group: Cereal grains furnish the bulk of the world food supply. The six main crops—wheat, rice, rye, oats, corn and barley—would provide enough grain, if shared out equally today, for each person in the world to have nearly six hundred pounds (270 kg) a year. Cereal and cereal products are high in carbohydrates and furnish approximately 50 percent of the calories consumed by the people of the world. The nutritional composition of various cereal grains is listed in Table 5.5. A cereal grain consists of three parts: the inner germ, the protective endosperm, and the outer bran layer. The germ or embryo of the grain is one of the best sources of thiamin and vitamin E. It also contains B-complex vitamins, fat, minerals (especially iron), carbohydrate and complete protein. Endosperm makes up approximately 85 percent of the grain and is chiefly car-bohydrate, with some protein in the form of gluten. The bran or outer layer, is chiefly cellulose (fiber) plus B-complex vitamins and minerals, especially iron. Whole grains include all three parts and provide significant amounts of iron, thiamin, riboflavin and niacin. Highly refined cereal grain products contain only the endosperm, and lack fiber and the natural minerals and vitamins. The consumption of whole grain products is, therefore, highly important to obtain the proper nutritional value of the bread and cereal group.

Protein Group

Nuts: Nuts are high in protein and fat, which makes them an important meat replacement for a vegetarian. The commonly used edible nuts are peanuts, almonds, walnuts, cashews, pecans, Brazil nuts, chestnuts, pistachios, filberts, hazelnuts, macadamias. The nutritional value of different nuts varies. Most are rich in protein; almonds 20 percent, cashews 17 percent, Brazil nuts 13 percent, walnuts 12 percent. Peanuts and pine nuts are even richer in protein. Peanuts may be 28 percent and pine nuts 31 percent protein. Nuts are delicious foods with natural flavors. However, you might have come across bitter almonds which are so bitter as to be inedible—fortunately so, since they contain a harmful substance called prussic acid. Since nuts are high in fat (except chestnuts), they digest slowly and help in delaying a feeling of hunger. Nuts are a good source of B-complex vitamins, thiamin, riboflavin and niacin and of the minerals iron, copper, pho-sphorus and manganese. They also contain varying amounts of calcium, depending upon the variety.

Legumes: High in food value and fine in flavor, legumes such as peas and beans come as near as possible to being perfect vegetables. Legumes supply important quantities of protein and are low in fat (see Table 5.5). As discussed earlier in this chapter, these can be used in combination with other foods such as cereal grains to provide a high quality protein. They are valuable in any diet and invaluable to vegetarians. There are many varieties of legumes, including lima beans, split peas, lentils, red kidney beans, pinto beans, mung beans, black-eyed peas, chickpeas and many others. Peas are the most successful of all frozen vegetables since they do not lose their vitamin C when frozen. In the process of canning, however, peas lose most of their vitamin C value. Dried beans and peas are bursting with protein—about 20 percent. It puts them on a par with meat; in fact they are better because of their low fat value as compared to meat. The same is true for the protein values of chickpeas and other legumes such as lentils. In addition to protein, legumes supply important quantities of iron, thiamin, riboflavin and trace minerals. Dried legumes lack vitamin C but by sprouting them they can be made rich in both C and B vitamins.

Fruit-Vegetable Group

Vegetables: All vegatables are good sources of minerals, vitamins and fiber. Selection of quality produce and careful adherence to proper food preparation technique are imperative in order to get the highest food value from vegetables. Nature provides the proper foods for the proper season, so try to use freshly harvested vegetables. Many families obtain fresh vegetables from a garden planted in the backyard. The nutritive value of frozen vegetables is equal to that of the fresh ones, but when vegetables are canned some nutritive elements are lost. Although many vegetables can be eaten raw, others require cooking which needs proper attention to retain the food values. As a general rule, the shorter time you cook most vegetables, the better. This does not refer to vegetables such as potatoes or squash which may be baked for a longer time if left whole in their skin. Many vitamins are water soluble. If vegetables are boiled in a lot of water and then the water is poured down the drain, much of the nutrition goes with it. One good method to cook vegetables such as carrots or beets is to grate them, put a small amount of oil in a sauce pan, add the grated vegetable, cover, and steam for about 3 minutes over a medium heat. Oil frying has an advantage of locking in the vitamins.

Vegetables may be classified according to the part of the plant used for food and according to nutritive value. Different parts of vegetables, like different vegetables, vary in nutritive value.

Green Leafy and Flowering Vegetables: Lettuce, romaine, chicory, cabbage, collards, Chinese cabbage, escarole, endive and all greens are examples of green leafy vegetables. Broccoli and cauliflower are the most commonly used flowering vegetables. Salad is one of the most popular vegetarian dishes in the West usually contains lettuce (the most popular salad plant) or a mixture of several raw green leaves. In many European countries salad is eaten with the main meal but in the United States it is often eaten at the start of a meal. The latter has an advantage in that you are likely to eat more health-promoting salad when you are hungry at the start of a meal. Eating salad helps to avoid the danger of obesity because salad is low in calories. Also the bulkiness of salad, and the time taken to eat it, lessen intake of more fattening food. Mixed salads often contain tomatoes, cucumber, beets and scallions in addition to lettuce and various other ingredients. Try to avoid dressing, but for taste lemon juice or vinegar along with a little salt and black pepper may be added.

On nutritional counts, green vegetables are most valuable in their amounts of minerals, vitamins and cellulose; they are important sources of the minerals calcium and iron and of the vitamins A, K and riboflavin, and they are valuable sources of vitamin C. The young, tender growing leaves contain more vitamin C than the mature plants. The carotene in green vegetables can be converted into vitamin A by the human body and the amount of carotene is more or less related to the amount of green pigment; therefore greener vegetables are richer in vitamin A. Among flowering vegetables, broccoli, being greener, rates higher in nutritive value than cauliflower and is a good source of iron, phosphorus, vitamin A, vitamin C and riboflavin. Cauliflower is also a good source of vitamin C; one half cup of cooked cauliflower contains about 70 mg. The leafy green and flowering vegetables are generally low in calories (Table 5.5).

Underground (Root and Tubers) Vegetables: Carrots, beets, turnips, radishes, rutabaga, kohlrabi, and parsnips are examples of root vegetables (modified roots), while potatoes, artichokes, and sweet potatoes are examples of tubers (modified underground stems). The yellow and orange varieties are rich sources of carotene. The deeper the yellow color, the greater the content of carotene, which is the precursor of vitamin A. The main positive virtue of most roots lie in their mineral content, but they also have value in their low-calorie bulk, so that they fill without fattening. There is also the likelihood that you will at least enjoy some of them, if not all, for their flavor. Radishes and beets, for example, are flavorful additions to green salads and contribute not more than 30 Calories per hundred grams. Carrots have the additional merit of being very rich in carotene, which the body converts into vitamin A. To ensure that this substance is not squandered, the carrots should not be deep scraped or peeled, for the greatest concentration of carotene is in the skin or just beneath it. Root vegetables in general are good sources of thiamin. Some have a moderate amount of vitamin C. Kohlrabi, for example, contains as much vitamin C as oranges. The underground stems or tubers, of potatoes, yams and artichokes provide a substantial amount of energy-giving starch. Sweet potatoes and artichokes have a sweeter taste than that of other tubers because they also contain some sugars. The caloric values of tubers are higher than root vegetables because of their higher carbohydrate content (see Table 5.5). Potatoes contain ascorbic acid, thiamin and niacin which can add significantly to daily allowance, if potatoes are properly prepared and consumed in sufficient quantity. The deep peeling of a potato results in a loss of up to a quarter of the potato's protein because protein is most highly concentrated just below the skin. If a peeled potato is boiled, up to half of its vitamin C content is dissolved in the cooking water. So to retain as much nutrients as possible, bake or boil unpeeled potatoes.

Stem or Stalk Vegetables: Celery and asparagus are common examples of stem vegetables. They contain minerals and vitamins in proportion to the green color, similar to that found in green leafy vegetables. Celery, being low in calories (Table 5.5) and good in taste, is most popular among people on a diet; its caloric values, in fact, are so low that digesting celery may use more energy than that provided by its nutrient contents. Asparagus contains a considerable amount of protein, a fair amount of ascorbic acid and is exceptionally rich in folic acid (member of vitamin B-complex).

Fruit Vegetables: The common examples of fruit vegetables are tomato, pepper, cucumber, squash, pumpkin, and eggplant; all of these are actually the fruit of a plant. Growing fat on fruit vegetables is unlikely because these contain more than 90 percent water, only the merest trace of fat, and very little carbohydrate. The avocado (which stands out among vegetables and fruit) is the exception and it contains 17 percent fat. Fruit vegetables have little caloric value, but our diet would be poorer without them. The fruit vegetable that excels all others in flavor is the tomato. Eaten raw it is a good source of carotene and vitamin C, and is low in calories; half a pound of raw tomatoes provides only 35 Calories. Peppers are another exceptionally good source of vitamin C. They contain about six times as much as tomatoes. Remember, the deeper the green or yellow color, the greater the carotene (precursor of vitamin A) content of a vegetable. Another fruit vegetable, cucumber is not nutritionally important but has a unique flavor when eaten raw or cooked. Although some people dislike cucumbers because they are hard to digest, the cucumbers can be made less indigestible by thinly slicing the unpeeled cucumber, sprinkling it with salt and then after about an hour pouring off the resulting liquid.

Bulb Vegetables: Onions and garlic are the most universally used and apparently the most indispensable vegetables. Possibly they make people feel good because onions are known to improve the circulation of the blood. It has now been discovered that onions reduce serum cholesterol, thus helping to lessen the likelihood of coronary heart disease. The onions are also known to stimulate natural contractions of the intestine. Nutritionally, onions are high in sulfur and a fair source of vitamin C. The old myths that onion juice rubbed on a bald head will grow hair or that onions cure boils, restore bad eyesight, reduce blood pressure, increase lust, clean out the bowels and induce sleep have not yet been substantiated by scientific evidence. Similarly, old claims for garlic include that it made peasants work harder and soldiers fight more stubbornly. Health-food literature still frequently gives the impression that garlic will cure all ills, arthritis among them.

Mushrooms: Mushrooms do not contain chlorophyll, the green pigment found in other plants, so, instead of converting inorganic substances into organic, as green plants do, these have, like animals, to feed on organic material. There are numerous varieties of edible wild mushrooms but whoever plans to eat wild mushrooms should have a first-rate field guide to distinguish between edible and poisonous species. As a safe alternative, mass-produced cultivated mushrooms are usually available throughout the year. Besides adding flavor to many dishes, mushrooms are a good source of niacin as well as potassium and phosphorus.

Fruit: An apple a day is supposed to keep the doctor away because apples, like fruits in general, provide energy through their carbohydrate content; they add roughage to the diet; and they are a good source of natural minerals and vitamins. Fruits in general contain very little protein and are practically fat free. Two exceptions to the fat rule are avocados (also mentioned earlier under fruit vegetables) and olives, both of which contain appreciable amounts of fat. Fruits vary widely in their carbohydrate content (see Table 5.5) and have a comparatively low caloric value when fresh. Dried fruit such as raisins and fruits canned with sugar have increased calories. Although all fruits contribute some ascorbic acid, the citrus fruits are outstanding as a source of this vitamin. For example, one medium-size orange will furnish the normal adult daily requirement. Fruits also supply varying amounts of vitamin A and the B-complex vitamins. The yellow fruits, such as peaches, cantaloupe and apricots are good sources of the pigment carotene, a precursor of vitamin A. Plums and dried fruits are the best sources of thiamin. Fruits in general contribute appreciable amounts of the minerals iron and calcium. Among the fruits richest in iron are dried fruits of all kinds (raisins, dates, dried figs, prunes) as well as apricots, peaches, bananas, grapes and berries. Calcium is found in citrus fruits, strawberries and dried figs. Dried figs are also high in fiber and protein as well as in B vitamins; their gentle laxative action adds to their health-giving properties. Sodium, magnesium and potassium are present in varying amounts in most fruits.

Careful preparation and storage of fruits are essential to retain the maximum value of vitamins and minerals. For example, clinical studies reveal that many children and adults do not get enough ascorbic acid even though the consumption of citrus fruits has increased greatly in the last century; this is due to lack of knowledge about its sources, preparation and storage, rather than to cost or availability. If peeling is required, for instance, fruit should be peeled thinly to conserve the nutrients. Fresh fruit should be chilled before the juice is extracted, which should be done just before serving. This is because bruising, cutting, and allowing fruit juice to be exposed to the air cause considerable loss of ascorbic acid. If juices are stored in a refrigerator, they should be put in covered containers (preferably air tight) to reduce oxidation and loss of vitamin C. The fruits which can be frozen compare favorably to fresh ones in nutritive value.

Milk Group: A breast-fed infant and a suckled calf are both getting their perfect food—mother's milk which is nature's way to perfect nutrition. Although the milk

Table 5.6 Nutrient content of cow's milk, human milk, and infant formula per liter.

Nutrient	Cow's milk	Human milk	Typical infant formula
Calories	670	750	680
Protein (gm) (Casein, Lactoalbumin)	36	11	16
Carbohydrate (gm) (Lactose)	49	68	72
Fat (gm)	36	45	36
Cholesterol (mg)	113	200	160
Vitamin A (I.U.)	1,447	1,898	2,500
Vitamin D (I.U.)	400	22	400
Vitamin E (I.U.)	1.5	2.7	15
Vitamin C (I.U.)	10	43	55
Folacin (microgram)	55	52	50
Niacin (milligram equiv.)	9.5	1.5	7.0
Riboflavin (mg)	1.8	0.36	1.0
Thiamin (mg)	0.3	0.16	0.6
Vitamin B_6 (mg)	0.5	0.1	0.4
Vitamin B_{12} (mg)	5.3	0.3	1.5
Vitamin K (microgram)	60	15	65
Calcium (mg)	1,220	340	510
Phosphorus (mg)	960	140	390
Iodine (microgram)	47	30	68
Iron (mg)	0.5	0.2	1.5
Magnesium (mg)	120	40	41
Zinc (mg)	4	1.6	5
Copper (microgram)	300	240	400
Sodium (milliequivalents)	22	7	10
Potassium (milliequivalents)	38	13	18
Chloride (milliequivalents)	28	11	15

SOURCES: Fomon, S. J. *Infant Nutrition*, W. B. Saunders Co., Philadelphia, 1974.
Composition of infant formulas from Ross Laboratories, Columbus, Ohio.
National Dairy Council, *Newer knowlege of milk*, 3rd ed. Chicago, 1972.

of all mammals has the same constituents, the proportion of constituents differs. For example, human milk contains less protein and more carbohydrate than cow's milk (Table 5.6). By any standard milk is still the most valuable of all foods in the human diet; it contains high-quality protein (mainly casein with small amounts of lactoalbumin and lactoglobulin), fat (cream), carbohydrate (lactose or milk sugar), the minerals calcium and phosphorus, and the vitamins riboflavin, niacin, vitamin A and (when the milk is fortified) vitamin D (see Table 5.6). The exact composition of milk varies to some degree with the breed of cattle, the season of the year, and the feed given to the animal.

Three-fourths of the calcium, nearly one-half of the riboflavin, and one-fourth of the protein, normally, come from milk in the average food supply. To keep calories and fat level down the use of skim or low-fat milk is quite effective. One pint of skim milk has 180 Calories as compared to one pint of whole milk which provides 320 Calories. Although milk is extremely important as a rich source of protein, minerals, and vitamins for a growing child, it is still necessary for adults and senior citizens as a source of calcium. Calcium in milk appears to be extremely important in delaying deossification or osteoporosis; a bone loss which results in weakening of skeletal strength, and the occurrence of fractures with just minimal stress. If milk is not liked as a beverage, it can be taken in the form of cheese or yogurt or used in various other dishes involving milk or milk products.

To make milk safe from any kind of pathogenic bacteria, most milk is pasteurized, even though this process destroys some of the thiamin and vitamin C. The pasteurization of milk involves heating milk to destroy pathogenic bacteria and then cooling it rapidly. If milk is not pasteurized, a home pasteurization (heating of milk until it comes to a boil) is generally useful. Certified milk is not pasteurized but must meet standards of cleanliness. Milk may also be homogenized, a process that reduces the size of the cream particles. As a result, the cream does not rise to the top of the milk but stays suspended throughout the liquid.

Cheese: Milk or cheese are one of the meat alternatives because of the similarity of nutrients, particularly animal proteins. The nutrients in cheese are more concentrated than in milk (Table 5.5), and cheese is an excellent source of protein and also of calcium, riboflavin and vitamin A. But with the exception of such low-fat cheeses as cottage cheese, it is also high in saturated fat and cholesterol. Thus, moderate consumption of cheese is wise, especially for those with heart problems. The type of milk used in the manufacture of cheese reflects the nutritive qualities of the cheese. For example, protein, calcium and vitamin B factors are contributed by the whole milk used in cheddar cheese—often called American cheese. Cottage cheese (unripened soft cheese) is less concentrated than cheddar cheese, with about four-fifths as much protein per pound.

Yogurt: Of all dairy foods, health food lovers rank yogurt as supreme. Yogurt is one of the oldest health foods. The ancient Hebrews ate yogurt, as did the Egyptians. In the book of *Genesis* there is a mention that Abraham ate yogurt and served it to his guests. Yogurt is a staple of the Bulgarians, who eat it daily and have one of the highest rates of longevity in the world. Yogurt is one food that has long been associated with the attainment of great age. Yogurt contains more protein and riboflavin than milk itself and is more easily digested.

Yogurt is a fermented milk product made from whole, low-fat or skim milk. The bacteria usually used are *Lactobacillus bulgaricus*, *Streptococcus thermophilus* and possibly *Lactobacillus acidophilus*. Yogurt retains all the food value of the milk from which it is made. Yogurt is not exceptionally low in calories unless it is made from skim milk and is unsweetened.

Natural Diet Plan to Getting Thin and Staying Thin—
Feel Healthy but not Hungry

As you know from the preceding pages, the natural diet containing whole foods of plant origin (except milk) is generally low in fat, cholesterol and caloric values, but high in stomach-filling bulk such as fiber, and in health-promoting natural vitamins and minerals. The following pages will include diet plans mainly as guidelines. Although these are confined for the most part to natural vegetarian foods, fat free lean meats and meat analogues (discussed earlier in this chapeter) may be included in small amounts as a supplement until you start enjoying exclusively vegetarian foods.

To follow the diet plan you can easily improvise your own menu for the day from the listed food groups in Table 5.7. As a rule of thumb, include foods from the first three groups varying from 1 to 4 servings (Table 5.7) depending on in-dividual weight status. Table 5.8 provides an example of how to select various food groups from Table 5.7 to choose a diet of 1,000 Calories which provides 53 grams of protein. For maximum weight loss with an intake of 600–700 Calories, choose one serving from group 1 and two from each of groups 2 and 3. From the vegetable and fruit groups 4 and 5 choose about 4 servings. In fact, the foods from groups 4, 5 and 6 are so low calorically that they can be eaten in relatively unlimited amounts. To keep from being hungry these unrestricted foods help the dieter avoid the temptation to deviate by providing a satisfying sense of bulk while adding very few calories.

Unless there is a serious weight problem, weighing of food is not necessary as long as you are eating plenty of natural food, particularly from groups 4 and 5 with the added taste of seasonings from group 6. As you may notice, the fat food group is not added. In addition to the natural fat provided by the food itself, most of the cooking requires frying in vegetable oils such as corn, cottonseed, safflower, soy, sunflower, olive and margarine which will provide enough fat.

A variety of vegetables used in suggested combinations and recipes provided in the appendix of this book can lead you to new interesting low-calorie dishes of excellent taste which can keep you slim and healthy for the rest of your life. How-ever, cooking vegetables requires a great deal of time in preparation for peeling, slicing, chopping, etc. You can cut down the time by cooking extra quantities for the freezer.

Unlike many diet books, sample menus are not provided here. Taste is a personal choice and, perhaps like you, I do not like someone to tell me what to eat. As long as you follow the guidelines to include foods from all the six groups mentioned in Table 5.7 with special emphases on groups 4 and 5, you do not have to count calories or follow any sample menus. Compulsively counting calories and rigidly following sample menus of foods you do not like is not a part of the natural diet philosophy.

Table 5.7 Food groups of various nutritional values.

Group 1. Dairy Products. One serving of milk or milk products contains 12 grams of carbohydrate, 8 grams of protein, a trace of fat and 80 Calories.

Dairy Product (Non-Fat Fortified)	Amount/serving
Skim or non-fat milk	1 cup
Powdered (non-fat dry, before adding water)	1/3 cup
Canned, evaporated skim milk	1/2 cup
Buttermilk made from skim milk	1 cup
Yogurt made from skim milk (plain, unflavored)	1 cup

Group 2. Grains and starchy vegetables. The amounts of one serving contain 15 grams of carbohydrate, 2 grams of protein and 70 Calories.

Food	Amount/serving
Bread	
Whole wheat	1 slice
Rye or pumpernickel	1 slice
Raisin	1 slice
Bagel, small	1/2
English muffin, small	1/2
Plain roll, bread	1
Frankfurter roll	1/2
Hamburger bun	1/2
Dried bread crumbs	3 tbsp
Tortilla, 6″	1
Cereal	
Bran flakes	1/2 cup
Other ready-to-eat unsweetened cereal	3/4 cup
Puffed cereal (unfrosted)	1 cup
Cereal (cooked)	1/2 cup
Grits (cooked)	1/2 cup
Rice or barley (cooked)	1/2 cup
Pasta (cooked) Spaghetti, noodles, macaroni	1/2 cup
Popcorn (popped, no fat added)	3 cup
Cornmeal (dry)	2 tbsp
Flour	2 1/2 tbsp
Wheat germ	1/4 cup
Cracked wheat cereal (cooked)	1/3 cup
Oatmeal (cooked)	1/3 cup
Brown rice (cooked)	1/3 cup
Starchy Vegetables	
Corn	1/3 cup
Corn on cob	1 small
Parsnips	2/3 cup
Potato, white	1 small
Potato (mashed)	1/2 cup
Pumpkin	3/4 cup
Winter squash, acorn or butternut	1/2 cup

Table 5.7 continued.

Food	Amount/serving
Yam or sweet potato	1/4 cup

Group 3a. Legumes. The amounts of one serving contain 20 grams of carbohydrate, 7 grams of protein, 1/2 gram of fat and 100 Calories.

Food	Amount/serving
Beans, peas, lentils (dried and cooked)	1/2 cup
Baked beans, no pork (canned)	1/4 cup
Lima beans	1/2 cup
Peas, green (canned or frozen)	1/2 cup

Group 3b. Meats. One exchange of lean meat (1 oz) contains 7 grams of protein, 3 grams of fat and 55 Calories. The meats here are selected for low in saturated fat.

Type	Amount/serving
Beef: Baby beef (very lean), chipped beef chuck, flank steak, round (bottom, top), all cuts rump, spare ribs, tripe	1 oz
Lamb: Leg, rib, sirloin, loin (roast and chops), shank, shoulder	1 oz
Pork: Leg, (whole rump, center shank), ham, smoked (center slices)	1 oz
Veal: Leg, loin, rib, shank, shoulder, cutlets	1 oz
Poultry: Meat without skin of a chicken, turkey, cornish hen, guinea hen, pheasant	1 oz
Fish: Any fresh or frozen	1 oz
Canned salmon, tuna, mackerel, crab and lobster	1/4 cup
Clams, oysters, scallops, shrimp	5 or 1 oz
Sardines (drained)	3

Group 4. Vegetables. One half cup serving of vegetables contains about 5 grams of carbohydrate, 2 grams of protein and 25 Calories. All vegetables are low calories non-fat, and exclude starchy vegetables.

Asparagus	Greens:
Bean sprouts	Mustard
Beets	Spinach
Broccoli	Turnip
Brussels sprouts	Mushrooms
Cabbage	Okra
Carrots	Onions
Cauliflower	Rhubarb
Celery	Rutabaga
Cucumbers	Sauerkraut
Eggplant	String beans, green
Green pepper	or yellow

Table 5.7 continued

Type	Amount/serving
Greens:	Summer squash
Beet	Tomatoes
Chard	Tomato juice
Collards	Turnips
Dandelion	Vegetable juice cocktail
Kale	Zucchini

The following raw vegetables may be used as desired:

Chicory	Lettuce
Chinese cabbage	Parsley
Endive	Radishes
Escarole	Watercress

Group 5. Fruits. The amounts of one serving of fruit contains 10 grams of carbo-hydrate and 40 Calories. All fruits listed are low calorie non-fat.

Fruit	Amount/serving
Apple	1 small
Apple juice	1/3 cup
Applesauce (unsweetened)	1/2 cup
Apricots, fresh	2 medium
Apricots, dried	4 halves
Banana	1/2 small
Berries:	
Blackberries	1/2 cup
Blueberries	1/2 cup
Raspberries	1/2 cup
Strawberries	3/4 cup
Cherries	10 large
Cider	1/3 cup
Dates	2
Figs, fresh	1
Figs, dried	1
Grapefruit	1/2
Grapefruit juice	1/2 cup
Grapes	12
Grape juice	1/4 cup
Mango	1/2 small
Melon:	
Cantaloupe	1/4 small
Honeydew	1/8 medium
Watermelon	1 cup
Nectarine	1 small
Orange	1 small
Orange juice	1/2 cup
Papaya	3/4 cup
Peach	1 medium

Table 5.7 continued

Fruit	Amount/serving
Pear	1 small
Persimmon, native	1 medium
Pineapple	1/2
Pineapple juice	1/3 cup
Plums	2 medium
Prunes	2 medium
Prune juice	1/4 cup
Raisins	2 tablespoons
Tangerine	1 medium

Group 6. Beverages and seasonings. The foods listed have no appreciable carbohydrate, protein or fat content if used in ordinary amounts.

Coffee	Rennet tablets
Tea	Celery seasoning
Clear broth	Cinnamon
Bouillion, without fat	Garlic
Gelatin, unsweetened	Lemon
Mint	Mustard
Nutmeg	Onion seasoning
Parsley seasoning	Pepper
Saccharin, Sucaryl and other	Vinegar
non-caloric sweeteners	Pickles (sour or unsweetened dill)

Table 5.8 Example for selecting a 1,000 Calorie diet from various food groups provided in Table 5.7.

Food Group	No. of servings	Calories	Protein (g)	Carbohy-drates (g)	Fat (g)
1. Dairy products	2	160	16	24	—
2. Grains and starchy vegetables	4	280	8	60	—
3. Legumes	3	300	21	60	5
4. Vegetables	No limit (4)	100	8	20	—
5. Fruits	No limit (4)	160	—	40	—
6. Beverages and seasonings	No limit	0	—	—	—
Total		1,000	53	204	5

A Few Simple Rules for Eating Habits

1. Always remember that we 'eat to live' and do not 'live to eat.'
2. Try to understand the nutritional values of food and—without becoming a diet freak—keep in mind the effects of various foods on your health.
3. Proper eating should be established, and regularly observed. However, do not eat just because it is meal-time unless you feel you need food.
4. Do not eat immediately before or after exercise or immediately after physical work or a hurried walk.
5. Do not involve yourself in hard mental work for at least 15 minutes before and after meals. If tired, relax for 10–15 minutes before eating. Pleasant conversation or relaxed thinking while eating is good; arguing or concentrating on the day's problems is harmful.
6. Drinking pure water with food helps digestion. However, cut down at meal-times; drink about half an hour before or after a meal. Fruit juices are best, but fresh made tea will cause no harm.
7. Occasional fasting is useful; if possible, once a month is suggested.
8. Cleaning the mouth before and after meals is a healthful habit and keeps teeth healthy.
9. The teeth are the proper organs of mastication, and every particle of food that requires mastication should be subjected to this operation. Proper mastication saves the stomach from an extra burden.
10. Slow eating is a good habit and food should be taken into the system no faster than it can be thoroughly communicated by the teeth.

Mastication and slow eating are considered desirable in promoting health because they help in digestion and also in weight loss by diminishing any sensation of abnormal appetite. Fruit, whole grains, and raw vegetables—essentials of a good vegetarian diet—take a lot more chewing than meat and white bread. Besides being important for healthy teeth, thorough chewing stimulates secretion of saliva and gastric juices, which aid digestion. Poor digestion results in a disordered stomach. It is interesting to note that earlier nutrition experts considered digestion of food to be as important a part of nutrition as nutritional values. A list of various foods and their digestion time is given in Table 5.9 which is based on an experiment of Doctor Beaumont on St. Martin, who had a unique opportunity to observe very accurately the time required for digestion through a fistulous opening into the stomach.

Emphasis on digestion of food seems curious to most westerners because their common high meat diets with low fiber content are easy to digest. However, in view of the fiber fad, digestion and upset stomach due to high fiber consumption can be a problem. Therefore, gradual increase of fiber intake only from natural foods (and not the added fiber) and proper mastication of these foods are stongly suggested. If you happen to use a mild alcoholic beverage at meal times, it can help in digesting high fiber foods. However, remember that excessive consumption of alcohol not only adds calories, but is also addictive.

Table 5.9   Time required for the digestion of various foods.

Food	Digestion time	
	Hours	Minutes
Apples—sweet, raw	1	50
sour, hard, raw	2	50
Barley, boiled	2	
Broiled rock fish	3	
Beans boiled in pod	2	30
Beans and green corn boiled (succotash)	3	45
Beef, roasted or boiled	3	
Beef, dried or salted, boiled	4	15
Beets, boiled	3	45
Bread made of wheat	3	30
Bread made of corn	3	15
Butter melted	3	30
Cabbage, raw	2	50
Cabbage in vinegar	2	
Cabbage, boiled	4	30
Cheese, old and strong	3	30
Chicken, stewed	2	45
Cod fish, dry, boiled	2	
Duck, roasted	4	
Eggs, hard boiled	3	30
Eggs, soft boiled	3	
Eggs, raw	2	
Goose, wild, roasted	2	30
Lamb, broiled	2	30
Liver, beef's broiled	2	
Meat and vegetables, hashed	2	30
Milk	2	
Mutton	3	
Oysters, raw	2	55
Oysters, stewed	3	30
Pork, roasted	5	15
Pork, stewed	3	
Potatoes, Irish, boiled	3	30
Potatoes, roasted, baked	2	30
Rice, boiled	1	
Sago	1	15
Salmon, salted	4	
Tapioca, boiled	2	
Tripe, boiled	1	
Trout, boiled	1	30
Turkey, boiled	3	55
Turnips, boiled	2	30
Veal, broiled	4	
Venison steak	1	35

SOURCE: Manual of Homeopathic Practice, 1855.

A Thought of Caution: Any individual reading about nutrition will generally pick up at least two things and most likely practice these: eat foods high in protein and take vitamins including mineral supplements every day. Even if one does not read about nutrition, one will learn from other sources such as television or other commercial media. People not only eat foods such as meats with high protein but also take protein concentrates in the form of tablets and liquid; they do the same with vitamins. Oddly enough, the manufacturers of nutritional supplements often appear to be trying to convince people that nearly everyone's diet is somehow unbalanced or inadequate and therefore in need of the supplements they sell. The recent fortification schemes are not responses to established nutritional needs so much as attempts to cash in on the new fad. Some 1.3 billion dollars are spent on nutritional supplements each year based on a simple philosophy of "if a little is good, more must be better."

I do not doubt any of the findings indicating important functions of proteins and vitamins as well as of other nutrients. Of course, some people do have deficiencies that should be corrected. Pregnant and nursing women, heavy drinkers, strict dieters, women taking oral contraceptives, and those who eat a limited variety of food may require supplemental vitamins and minerals. But most circumstances that compromise vitamin and mineral nutrition can be managed through diet rather than supplements. For example, there is evidence that heavy smokers and persons undergoing surgery might benefit from extra vitamin C, which can be easily obtained by eating more C-rich foods.

Although vitamins and minerals used in large quantities as drugs have proved useful in combating certain medical disorders, controversies over benefits and risks of large doses still exist. The fad of nutritional supplements certainly should be treated with caution at the current state of knowledge. We have already realized some of the problems which are caused by the use of concentrated nutrients and by moving away from natural foods. Some examples (details emphasized in appropriate sections of this book) are, diseases related to lower fiber content, uric acid problems, saturated fats in meat, overweight and diseases related to obesity, and so on.

Excessive vitamins taken as supplements are either excreted from the body, stored in body fat and other organs, or used by the body as drugs to perform other, non-vitamin functions. It is the body buildup or storage of the excess that often causes serious side effects. Vitamins A, D, E, and K are especially risky in large amounts because, as fat-soluble vitamins, they are stored in the body. Too much D can cause kindney stone, irreversible kidney damage, abnormal heart rhythms, lethargy, and coma. Excessive amounts of vitamin E can interfere with blood clotting. Although the most popular vitamin, vitamin C, is not stored in the body because it is water-soluble, nonetheless, excessive quantities can create a dependency; when intake is suddenly discontinued, deficiency symptoms such as scurvy may appear. The Food and Drug Administration (FDA) advisory panel in March 1979 evaluated and recommended that vitamin K, copper, fluoride, iodine, magnesium, manganese, phosphorus and potassium not be sold in megadose quantities as drugs; their recommendations, however, have yet to be put into effect. As a simple rule, almost any substance—including water—can have harmful, indeed fatal, side effects if consumed in great enough quantities.

Meanwhile, in the face of nutritional controversies, in order to avoid any of the known or still unknown risks, a safe practice is to follow a natural diet accompanied by nutritional knowledge. When we consume vitamins from natural foods they are (1) not concentrated, (2) accompanied by other food nutrients to share metabolic reactions, (3) associated with their natural solvents (e.g. nuts with oil and oil soluble vitamins). Moreover, our knowledge about the functioning of the body and about nutrients is still not complete. There are thousands of research articles and new findings appearing every year. Nature is wise and has helped us in our existence for thousands of years. A good idea, then, is to stick with nature's natural foods and use the scientific knowledge (gained by the efforts of many fine minds) to select the foods we eat.

Note: Food faddism is a term of concern that needs to be wiped out. Health professionals are now in general agreement that food faddists are not those who eat raw broccoli, wheat germ, and yogurt, but those who start the day on breakfast squares, gulp down bottle after bottle of soda pop, and snack on candy and twinkies (Jacobsen, 1975, *Nutr. Action*, Vol. 2, p. 1).

Vegetarians are sometimes called "food faddists," although vegetarianism certainly is not a food fad; as discussed in this Chapter, carefully planned vegetarian diets can be balanced, adequate, and can even offer nutritional benefits that are not characteristic of the typical American diet. Vegetarian diets are usually lower in total saturated fat, calories, total fat, and cholesterol and are higher in dietary fiber. Strict vegetarians have been found to average 20 lb less in body weight than nonvegetarians, who averaged 12 to 15 lb above their ideal weight. The same study found that pure vegetarians had significantly lower serum cholesterol levels (Hardinge and Stare, 1954, *J. Clin. Nutr.*, Vol. 22, p. 73). However, careful planning and nutritional knowledge to aid the vegetarian, to include the variety and appropriate combinations of food is essential (as discussed in this Chapter).

Many users of health foods are extreme in their search for clean, healthful, and uncontaminated food. Examples of these health food users are those who adhere to extreme forms of the Zen macrobiotic diet, those who consume huge quantities of vitamin/mineral supplements, those who depend on large amounts of "body-building" high-protein supplements, and those who subsist on only a few foods. As you have noticed in this Chapter, natural diet is not any one of these. Many young people, students, concerned mothers, and homemakers favor the use of health foods, and their diets are much "healthier" today than the average American diet. Wolff (Wolff, 1975, *Am. J. Clin. Nutr.*, Vol. 2, p. 116) suggests that these individuals, who are sometimes called food faddists should be called "health foodists." The term health foodist refers to those who have realistic ideas about nutrition and are seriously concerned about promoting health through eating good food.

Chapter 6

Slow Down Aging to Lead a Long and Healthy Life

All the pages of this book on health and happiness are in reality devoted to leading a long and healthy life. In this chapter, emphasis will be placed specifically upon markers of aging, aging theories, and hints for slowing down the aging process to prolong the enjoyment of good health. In addition to necessary individual efforts towards this end, it is possible that future research directed towards a basic understanding of the aging process may help to prolong life, perhaps not only by decades but multiples of decades. If hints in this chapter result in a younger appearance, this appearance will not be skin-deep (as achieved by cosmetics), but will stem from deep-down improvements in health. In other words, the point is not only to look younger but to feel younger.

Biological Markers of Aging

According to the National Institute on Aging, biological markers of aging are those physical and behavioral changes that occur at predictable times during the aging process. The identification of these biological markers is important in order to test any agents or methods designed to change the rate of aging. In this chapter, some of the biological markers are used to indicate the scientific validity of ancient breathing and yogic claims (as discussed in next two chapters) to maintain youthful health.

In humans, some predictable aging markers include decline in lung capacity and chest expansion, decrease in pupil size, bone loss, sleep variations, alterations in glucose tolerance and immune function, cardiovascular changes, and loss of specific hearing and vision.

Decreased Lung Function: Decreased lung capacity and chest expansion is one of the best indicators of declining health and or aging. These parameters which reflect forced vital capacity (FVC) determine the volume of air one can expel after taking a deep breath. The vital capacity, which is independent of sex, weight, and smoking habits, appears to decline steadily with age in both sexes, falling about 3.8 deciliters per decade in men and 3.1 deciliters per decade in women. The reasons are not clear, but it seems to be related more to chest wall function than to intrinsic factors in the lung function. Other indicators related to decline in breathing capacity show that older adults breathe with greater difficulty and less satisfaction than in earlier years. Past 40 years of age the basal metabolic rate (oxygen consumption) slowly declines until about 80 years of age when a very rapid decline is noted. As a result of decline in metabolic rate, the older people get tired easier (as we normally notice). The breathing exercises and yoga emphasized in Chapters 7 and 8 improve breathing efficiency, as well as lung capacity and chest expansion. This would tend to support the claim that breathing exercises and yoga maintain youthful health and improve vigor and vitality.

Pupil Size: Studies of the age-related contraction of the pupil have indicated that as we age, changes in pupil and lens reduce the light available to our retina. The retina of a 20-year-old person may be receiving three times as much light as the retina of 40-year-old. Moreover, the speed of adjustment to light change also declines with increasing age—in addition to reduced illumination due to smaller pupil size. Robert Sekuler and his colleagues from Northwestern University in Illinois found in a study on 120 volunteers ranging in age from 21 to 81 that on average, the subjects age 55 or over had 3 mm pupils and younger than 55 had 4 mm pupils. It is not known why pupil size decreases with advancing age. The possible causes may include atrophy of the dialater muscle fibers, deposition of a hyaline substance below the iris sphincter muscles, and loss of photoreceptors feeding the pupillary light reflex.

Farsightedness is another vision-related functional change generally associated with age. Many people need glasses when they approach age 40 to 45. The reason for a decreasing ability to focus on near objects with advancing age probably results from changes in the lens and the muscular forces acting upon it.

Bone Loss: Decrease in bone mass is probably responsible for the bulk of fractures in the older people. Peak bone mass (maximum cortical thickness and cross sectional area) is reached sometime between age 30 and 40, thereafter, loss occurs slowly, averaging 0.3% per year. It is the peak bone mass which determines the risk for fracture at old age. The peak bone mass, however, is determined by genetic, mechanical, and nutritional factors and it varies in different individuals. Therefore, the risk of fracture due to bone loss is variable in different people depending upon their bone mass.

The cause of age-related bone loss is not certain and is perhaps due to decline in physical activity, decline in muscle mass, and decline in imposed mechanical loads on the skeleton. Bone loss caused by longterm bedrest and weightlessness, which may be repairable by assuming physical activity, indicates that keeping up the physical activity is a helpful hint to slow down this age-related problem. Increase in the calcium intake (e.g. by drinking milk as discussed in Chapter 5) is extremely helpful in delaying bone loss.

Sleep Variations: Sleep parameters that show a substantial change with age include time spent in bed, total sleep time and number of arousals after sleep onset. Studies show that older people spend more time at night lying in bed without being able to sleep. They also spend more time during the day in bed resting or napping than younger subjects do. The studies on total sleep time among older people are conflicting. However, the number of awakenings is clearly higher in older than young people. Researchers have found that many awakenings are due to breathing disturbances among healthy, elderly individuals. The importance of breathing (Chapter 7) again comes into the picture here as a component of youthful health. Very little research has been conducted on biological rhythms in human adults as a function of age, an area of possible great interest.

Major Physical Changes: The changes listed below do not require detailed emphasis, and are self-explanatory. These in fact are all too familiar to most of us.

1. Loss of stature or reduction in height
2. Increased weight
3. Loss of hair and/or grey hair
4. Complexion changes and changed appearance of the skin
5. Increased wrinkles
6. Diminished size of muscles and increased amount of fatty tissue and/or loose skin
7. Loss of teeth

Other Markers of Aging: Impairment of hearing with advancing age ranks second only to arthritis. The most common source of hearing deficiency is suggested to be a progressive bilateral loss of hearing (presbycusis) for tones and speech due to degenerative physiological changes in the auditory system. Other biomarkers of aging include changes in immune function, glucose intolerance, amino acid racemization, cardiovascular function, the autonomic nervous system, and psychomotor indices, discussed at the National Institute on Aging conference, Bethesda, Maryland in 1981.

There is no doubt that delaying death is one thing which can have the support of almost every adult in the world. People go through pain and expense to tighten a sagging skin, cover a balding scalp, color the grey. But prolonged life without the benefits of youth and health is not a sufficient achievement. Demand for long life and youthful health actually go back even before the Greek and Roman Empires ruled the world. "When the Greek Goddess of dawn, Eos, begged Zeus to bestow immortality upon her lover, Tithonus, she neglected to ask that he be granted eternal youth as well. So Tithonus grew older and older, yet could not die. Finally out of pity, Eos changed him into a grasshopper." Today in the twentieth century we are still exploring ways to extend the vigorous and productive years of life, and perhaps the best move at this time is to combine the ancient Eastern approaches with modern Western approaches, as emphasized throughout this book.

The Causes of Aging

Our bodies are made up of cells that number in the billions. The energy we use to perform any action is generated by metabolic reactions of individual cells. The cells are born, they multiply, they age, they die. One of the most prominent notions in experimental gerontology (science of aging) has been that organisms including ourselves age because cells age. What causes cells to become senescent or aged, however, is still an open question, confronting various theories.

Let us consider first the popular *genetic theory of aging*. Among other things, cells contain nucleic acids, namely DNA (deoxyribonucleic acid) and RNA (ribonucleic acid). Working together, these nucleic acids are fundamental to the life process. DNA in the nucleus tells RNA on the periphery how to build particular enzyme-proteins to carry out necessary functions of the cell. High-quality, undamaged DNA will produce good RNA and this in turn results in peak functioning of the cell, which provides energy and vitality to the organism. As we age, the quality of these nucleic acids deteriorates. There is a DNA repair system built into each cell. If, however, the damage to DNA is too subtle for the DNA repair system to detect, or if it accumulates faster than the repair system functions, the cell will gradually become defective in essential control systems or enzymes. This situation will be particularly serious for cells that do not divide after they have differentiated to their mature forms. These include brain and muscle cells. If such cells function poorly or die, they are not replaced. Nucleic acid damage may be less serious for dividing cells such as those of the liver or the lining of the gastro-intestinal track, because the process of dividing provides a constant source of new cells. Age-related damage of DNA in both animals and plants is reported in many recent studies including our own work. According to genetic theory, therefore, aging is due primarily to the damage of DNA, and thus slowing down aging means keeping the DNA healthy, as discussed later in this chapter.

Aging, according to the second prominent *free radicals theory*, is caused by free radicals and oxidative processes. You might have heard about this theory in relation to vitamin E, which is associated with energy and potency. Actually vitamin E is an antioxidant which interferes with reactions mediated by free radicals and oxidation reactions. Free radicals are missing an electron. For this reason, they are highly reactive entities, which can damage both DNA and other cell structures. Free radicals may either be produced by cells as a result of their metabolic processes or they may come from the environment. For example, eating foods which have been exposed to X-rays, cosmic rays and nuclear fallout could carry free radicals into our body. The use of X-ray to sterilize foods for storing (as shown on ABC television network "Good Morning America," 1981) should be considered with caution. The claim that use of X-ray is similar to exposing foods to heat is true. However, the possibility of free radicals having been formed during the exposure period cannot be ruled out. Free radicals can also be formed by direct exposure of body tissue to radiation. Damage by free radicals to DNA or other cell structures may be caused directly by reacting promiscuously with other molecules, causing them to become free radicals too, or indirectly by generating strong oxidizing agents. The oxidation of a molecule causes it to become less efficient or actually harmful. This, according to the free radical-oxidation theory, is the root cause of aging. As pointed out earlier, vitamin E, because it is an antioxidant, slows down oxidation and hence is thought to retard aging.

Support for the involvement of free radicals and vitamin E therapy in aging has come from the studies of L. Packer, University of California, Berkeley, and J. R. Smith, Veterans Administration Hospital, Martinez, California. They added vitamin E to cultured fibroblasts from human embryos which normally divide about 50 times. But in the presence of vitamin E, the cells continued to divide and to have youthful characteristics for about 120 population doublings; after that they too became senescent and died. The concentration of the vitamin E in the enriched culture medium was approximately the same as that in serum *in vivo*.

Another interesting theory of aging is the *crosslinkage theory of aging*, which emphasizes the effects of doubled or tripled molecules of protein. According to this theory, protein molecules, which are long chains of amino acids, become linked with other protein molecules. These doubled or tripled molecules of protein are unnatural to the body and they gum up the cells with useless endangering debris. In addition to crosslinkage between protein molecules, crosslinkage between DNA molecules also forms a part of the theory. When crosslinkages form between the strands of DNA, they can interfere with the functioning of DNA in ways discussed as part of the genetic theory of aging.

Still another popular theory of aging, *autoimmune aging*, suggests that with age some alterations occur in the body's immunological defense reaction, and the host attacks its own kind. As you know, the body's immune system protects it from disease and cancer. The major components of the immune system are two types of white blood cells, B cells and T cells. The main job of the B cells is to fight bacteria and virus attacks by releasing proteins called antibodies. The main job of the T cells is to attack and destroy cells foreign to the body, such as cancer cells and transplant cells. Dr. R. Walford of UCLA suggests that T cells malfunction with age, and as a result cancer increases as people get older because the T cells no longer vigorously attack cancer cells. Another result is that B and T cells behave abnormally, attacking not only disease organisms and cancer cells, but the body's own normal, healthy cells. This destruction of the body by its own protective immune system, as stated above, is called autoimmunity.

The spleen, which is a reservoir for red blood cells, protects the body during an accident. It is also a reservoir for the T cells which protect against invasion by foreign cells. Dr. T. Makinodian of the National Institute on Aging, showed that removal of the spleen increased life span in mice. He suggests that this result is due to the fact that T cells in older individuals can become defective and cause autoimmune aging. However, the spleen is still required because some of the functional T cells would be needed to fight disease and cancer cells. Dr. Makinodian further modified his experiment to determine that transfusion of T cells from the young animals could prolong age and fight disease.

It has also been suggested that autoimmune aging can be slowed or reversed by the use of thymosin, a hormone produced by the thymus which may be responsible for maintaining the function of T cells.

Removal of the spleen or use of a hormone thymosine are still too much in the experimental stage to be applied in prolonging human life. However, following a diet to slow autoimmune aging is practical, as will be discussed later in this chapter.

Other theories of aging include breakdown of the brain pacemaker, damage of cell membranes, loss of collagen elasticity, and so on. As you see, none of the theories (based on individual experiments) are conclusive and aging perhaps is a result of several factors that influence body functioning. The vagueness and experimental stage of these theories limit their immediate practical value. The best we can do is to use some of the practical hints provided by the aging theories. The dependable solution that has been supported by scientific evidence, as well as ancient experiences, is the protection of health from deterioration. The common causes of damage to cells due to stress, poor nutrition, improper breathing and exercise practices, however, are well established and known to most of us. Fortunately, these damages can be considerably reduced, by following good nutritional habits along with physical and mental activity as emphasized in this book.

Safe Practices to Slow Down Aging

As we have learnt, none of the age-related findings present a miracle solution to slow down the aging process—not yet at least. In fact the nature of theories is such that it is difficult to practice any particular method for slowing down the process of aging. The hints based on experimental evidence of certain theories, as well as on common sense ideas, are presented below that may be used to supplement the overall health approach.

Vitamin E and C: The free radical-oxidation theory of aging would suggest the use of antioxidants to slow down the damaging processes in the cells of the body, caused by free radicals and oxidation. Using vitamin E in order to feel young is a familiar idea to most of us. Since vitamin E and vitamin C are antioxidants, the theory would suggest that a simple and safe precaution to slow free radical and oxidation related damage would be to take vitamin E and C regularly. How much of these vitamins should be taken daily to slow down aging is an open question. The amounts of these vitamins used by Dr. Linus Pauling (Nobel Laureate in Chemistry and Peace) include 2 grams of vitamin C and 1,200 units of vitamin E, which are more than thirty times the U.S. recommended daily allowances. However, in the absence of specific data, a lower amount would be safer: not more than 500 mg (half a gram) of vitamin C and 300 units of vitamin E. Too much of an antioxidant can interfere with a cell's oxidation reactions and might impair the cell's functioning in some vital way.

Selenium, present in trace amounts in a wide variety of foods, seems to have an important antioxidant role, although it is not tested in humans. Other antioxidants such as BHT (used by the food industry to preserve freshness of stored foods) and ethxyquin have been shown to prolong the life of laboratory animals up to 25 percent higher than average. However, these at present are not considered safe for human consumption in amounts proportional to those used in animal experiments. Still, they offer support to the general theory that the use of antioxidants may serve as a possible method for life extension.

Lowering Polyunsaturated Fats in the Diet: Polyunsaturated fat is one of the substances which is more easily oxidized than others and thus gives rise to more free radical reactions, presumably, therefore, promoting aging due to free radical mediated damage to cells. Polyunsaturated fat has long been recommended as a replacement for saturated fats in order to reduce cholesterol in the blood, yet according to Dr. Harman of the University of Nebraska, College of Medicine, all dietary fat, not just saturated fat, should be limited. He found that increased amounts of polyunsaturated fats in the diet of mice decreased their life span, which he hypothesized was due to increased levels of free radical reactions. At this point, the lesson is that a lowered intake of fat, whether saturated or unsaturated, is nutritionally healthful.

Dieting to Slow Autoimmune Aging: One of the life-lengthening effects of dietary restriction, according to Dr. R. Walford of UCLA, is due to its slowing the rate of autoimmune aging. As discussed earlier, during age-related development of autoimmunity, the body fails to recognize its own cells and attacks and damages them. The prolongation of life induced by dietary restriction, Dr. Walford claims, is due to the fact that the immune system is more susceptible than any other body system to starvation. Dietary restriction does not seem to harm the immune system, instead it slows its harmful effect of attacking the body's own cells. In any case, restricting our diets by eating less, but maintaining adequate amounts of nutrition is healthy and can thus increase the life expectancy. The statistical data also supports that average or lower body weight up to 20 pounds increases the life expectancy as compared to overweight, and the restriction of diet in rats has been shown to increase their life spans up to 25 percent. The beneficial effects of lower weight to reduce the chances of heart diseases as well as the chances of diabetes, nephritis, cerebral hemorrhage, and various diseases of the digestive system are fairly well known.

Nucleic Acid Therapy: The genetic theory of nucleic acid damage with age gives rise to the suggestion that a diet rich in nucleic acids can not only prevent but also repair such damage. This might make cells function as efficiently as cells in younger individuals. Dr. Benjamin Frank of New York has claimed recovery of his patients from degenerative diseases by keeping them on a diet which was rich in DNA and RNA content. Although this is as yet quite speculative, there is definitely no harm in using this therapy and we can make a routine habit of eating foods which provide one to one and a half grams of nucleic acids per day. Patients with gout disease should, however, be careful because they cannot metabolize the amounts of purine provided by such a diet.

Since nucleic acids as such are not studied as nutrients, nutritionists do not have data on nucleic acid contents of foods. Perhaps findings such as those mentioned above may lead to more nutritional studies being directed towards this approach. Based on various sources, including our own studies, some general guidelines for a choice of foods rich in nucleic acids are provided below. You are probably accustomed to most of the foods. The proper distribution of these foods in a weekly diet would provide an average daily intake of one to two grams of nucleic acids in dietary form. Among meats, good sources of nucleic acids include sardines, salmon, non-vertebrate seafood (such as shrimp, lobster, clams, oysters), any kind of fish, and liver meats (e.g. chicken liver, beef liver). As pointed out above, a diet high in meat, especially the one containing higher amounts of nucleic acids, is believed to raise the uric acid level associated with a common gout disease. Therefore, plenty of fluids including water and fruit or vegetable juices should be used with a nucleic acid diet. Foods more appropriate to vegetarian diets, such as pinto and other beans, lentils, peas, asparagus, mushrooms, and spinach, are high in nucleic acids and should be included in the daily diet in accordance with individual eating habits. Vegetarian foods are also low in fat and cholesterol, and as compared to meats, the danger of uric acid level increase is also low. The germinating seeds of soybeans, for example, can provide about twice the amounts of nucleic acids as compared to dry seeds containing the same nutritional value. Thus, the sprouts which are generally associated with health foods are a good source of nucleic acids. As a rule of thumb, actively growing plant parts—in which cells are dividing and therefore DNA is being synthesized—are high in nucleic acids.

Some Common Healthy Activities to Slow Aging: Researchers in the field of gerontology support the positive effect of the following life activities on our health and aging.

1. Since a high stress environment is dangerous to health and longevity, the practice of mental approaches to reduce stress as emphasized in Chapter 2 are the most effective and safe way to control stress, and have been proven effective for centuries.
2. An active life—having a reason for living—can prolong life.
3. An active sex life, in general, is suggested to prolong youthful health. In healthy old men, the sex hormone testosterone has been observed at levels similar to those of younger men and sexual activity is related to hormonal level. Which comes first—the hormone level or the active sex life—researchers have yet to determine. Observation on people over sixty have indicated that men and women do not lose their physical capacity for sexual performance in terms of erection and orgasm; and sex experts believe that sexual activity helps to preserve sexual functioning and youthful feelings.
4. Good marriage and social life can prolong life. For example, married couples live longer than single people with an otherwise similar social life. These effects may be due in part to reduced stress as compared to lonely people.
5. Mental exercises such as reading and crossword puzzles, and physical aerobic exercises for about 15 minutes, three times a week can go a long way towards preserving the body and mind. However, exertion can actually shorten lifespan. So the message is to *do* but don't *overdo*.
6. Seven guidelines, some of which are familiar to us, have been suggested by

various health experts to prolong life. These include no smoking, moderate weight, moderate drinking, physical activity, eating breakfast, regular meals, and sleeping seven or eight hours—but not less than six or more than nine.

In the overall conclusion, safe habits to prolong life include proper nutrition, a diet rich in fiber, and low in animal fat, sugar and refined foods, as discussed in Chapter 5. Certain aging theories suggest a possible role for the regular use of vitamins E and C and foods rich in nucleic acids as another nutritional aspect of long and healthy living. However, some of the ideas of the Eastern world such as yogic breathing for vigor and vitality, postures to keep youthful body flexibility, and the effect of mind on our health and performance, as discussed elsewhere in this book, are very important for healthy and youthful living. These ideas of the Eastern world that are based on centuries of experience, are certainly safe and effective as compared to the modern aging theories which are still in the exploration stage.

Some Interesting Prescriptions to Slow Aging

The search for a way to restore youth and vigor and to extend life is man's oldest quest, the mystery that has tantalized him for centuries. Egyptians and Romans ate garlic in large quantities to lengthen life and increase strength. Many early Europeans tried youth-regaining remedies such as roots of the mandrake plant (belonging to the potato family) and even insects such as the Spanish fly.

Among the most popular youth-regaining remedies were the transplant or extracts of healthy sexual organs of animals such as monkey and goat testicles as a form of rejuvenation therapy. The rejuvenation therapy by injecting with cells from fetal animals was pioneered by a Swiss Doctor Paul Niehans who made a fortune by treating wealthy and often famous senior citizens. Among other remedies are, the lowering of body temperature in certain experimental animals to slow aging. Shots of the anesthetic procaine called Gerovital (made up of procaine hydrochloride and haematoporphyrin) has been claimed to help elderly patients regain youthful characteristics such as improved memories, muscular strength and skin texture. Still other suggestions that have been made to slow down aging are hormone preparations, lipofuscin inhibitors, lysosome membrane stabilizers and cross-link inhibitors. However, the uses of the above youth-promoting techniques in the absence of data and scientific validity are extremely dangerous, even if we ignore the possibility of long-term side effects. Clearly, getting the right food into our bodies along with moderate adherence to safe health practices which are backed up by some scientific validity is a good start towards health and longevity.

Future of Aging Research and Concluding Remarks

Genetic engineering has opened the possibility of transferring specific genes including the ones involved in aging, via bacterial plasmid or virus DNA. But in order to transfer a specific gene, we must learn the location and function of each gene (30,000 estimated in a human cell) along the DNA double helix inside the center of every cell. Genetic mapping to study gene locations has progressed in the last decade and it is only a question of time until every chromosome will be known to contain the genes for specific enzymes. The map once completed, can provide geneticists with a catalogue of genes which can be used in genetic engineering. So, if aging is a function of certain specific genes and/or the result of genetic breakdown, it may ultimately be possible to transplant new genes that would enable older people to regain the level of vitality they had during youth.

How far we are from actually applying genetic engineering to stop aging is a difficult prediction to make. Although the technology is developing very rapidly, research dealing with living organisms is not always straightforward. The important thing is that you do not have to wait for this genetic revolution or any other medical breakthrough. The important points emphasized in this chapter and elsewhere in the book to slow down aging process and to feel healthy are based primarily on natural diet and health care. Therefore, simple, safe, and practical hints exist for you to test for yourself.

Note: Gerontology (study of aging) is one of the most interdisciplinary branches of biology. Biochemists, for example, explore the ways in which protein, such as collagen alter their properties as the organism ages; zoologists and botanists investigate aging as a population phenomenon and speculate on its evolutionary significance; geneticists examine the effects of experimental alteration of genetic material on the aging process. Gerontologists have counted about 200 independent theories which try to explain the aging process. There is opportunity for scientists to speculate and test the various theories. Therefore, the fundamental research into aging could be the most suitable subject for inclusion in research institutions. The organizations in the United States, such as National Institute of Health has made possible the development of cautious proposals for the prevention or delay of major human disorders that may influence aging. However, inspite of worldwide efforts on basic aging research, the information is not yet complete, and considerably more basic research is needed. Although some authors (not research professionals) have tried to exploit the basic information and have suggested the use of high doses of chemicals tested in laboratory experiments, self-experimentation with anti-aging therapies may be dangerous and may shorten rather than lengthening the life span.

S. Fulder of the National Institute of Medical Research, London, states that efforts to improve the health can prolong the life span, which is possible to achieve by relatively simple methods. These methods are already known before the advent of experimental gerontology. Techniques such as yoga, taking exercise, the ingestion of wholesome but frugal diet, and of herbs and vitamins have all been reliably acknowledged to prolong the life span and to protect the body from degenerative diseases (S. J. Fulder, 1976, *Science and Culture*, Vol. 42, p. 86). However, this does not mean that aging research has not helped; experimental gerontology has added many possibilities (discussed in this Chapter), such as using antioxidants, vitamins E and C.

Chapter 7

Complete Breathing for Vigor and Vitality

One of the most important factors in our energy production is breath. As oxygen enters the body, it provides the fundamental fuel for the metabolic activities of the cells. The energy supplied by the respiratory process affects the functioning of our brain, our stamina, and our basic physical well-being.

$$Food + Oxygen \rightarrow Energy + Carbon\ dioxide + Water$$

Biologically, the process of respiration involves a series of chemical reactions that are completed through two major pathways, *glycolysis* and *Krebs cycle*. The major purpose of these series of reactions is to provide energy along with waste carbon dioxide and water by burning food in the presence of oxygen. The cells harness energy from food (carbohydrates, fats, proteins) by combining ADP (adenosine diphosphate) and phosphate to reform the energy-rich compound ATP. This energy captured by the ATP molecule powers the various biological functions of the body. Because the delivery and utilization of oxygen are crucial with respect to energy metabolism, the breath that provides oxygen is often called *vital breath* or *vital energy* (as used in this chapter).

The increase in oxygen intake during breathing can result from an increase in the depth (tidal volume) or in the rate of breathing, or both. At rest, the breathing rate is about 14 breaths per minute (breathing is faster in children, and still faster in infants) and the tidal volume averages 0.5 liter of air per breath. Thus the amount of air breathed per minute would be 7 liters (14×0.5 liter). However, exercise and breathing practices can significantly increase the amount of breathed air. In well-conditioned endurance athletes, the air intake may increase to 160 to 220 liters per minute in response to maximum metabolic demands. Breathing exercises, as compared to strenuous physical exercises, have the advantage of providing energy without physical exertion. Moreover, breathing exercises teach the full utilization of the lungs, emphasizing depth rather than rate of breathing. In general, most people breathe in a shallow manner and use their lungs at less than one-third of their full capacity. To correct this, breathing that uses the respiratory system to its optimum potential is required, letting as much oxygen into the body as possible while removing as much waste carbon dioxide as possible.

Breath control is an integral part of training the physical body and mind to increase energy and relieve stress. The mind and body are the instruments through which we receive all the experiences. The inter-connection between breathing, mind, and the body are proved by our daily experiences. When one is sitting idle, breathing slows down. Suspension of mental activity increases in proportion to the slowing down of the breath; in cases of asphyxia (unconsciousness caused by too little oxygen and too much carbon dioxide in the blood), mental activity ceases altogether until respiration is restored. On the other hand, if we are tense or afraid, our breathing becomes quick and shallow. The regulation of harmonized breath helps an individual to achieve regulation and steadiness of mind. Conversely, by controlling the mind, the vital breath that provides energy is also controlled.

When we concentrate and consciously regulate our breathing we are able to store up in our various nerve centers and brain a greater amount of vital energy. One who has abundant vital energy radiates vitality and strength, which can be felt by those coming in contact with him. The great prophets and saints had been suggested to have a control of vital energy, which gave them tremendous will power that brought thousands toward them and made them think as the prophets.

All the functions of vital energy will have to be learned and mastered slowly and gradually. With proper training, one can discover that there is an unequal supply of vital energy in various parts of the body. The feelings will become so subtle that mind can feel where there is a decreased supply of vital energy and possess the power to supply it.

Importance of Vital Breathing

To breathe means to live and to live means to breathe. Every living thing depends upon breathing and cessation of breathing is cessation of life itself. We constantly drain our life force or vital energy (ATP molecule, in biological sense) by our thinking, willing, acting, or motion of muscles. Since all of these activities use up the life force, constant replenishing is necessary, which can be accomplished primarily through breathing. Whoever practices breathing regularly and systematically can feel in his own body the great effect of vital energy.

When one inhales, he is producing vital energy by absorbing oxygen to increase metabolism. In the practice of breathing, the mind plays a great role and it is important to observe consciously everything that takes place in the phenomenon of breathing. There are people everywhere, who consciously or unconsciously have control over the vital breath or energy. These spiritualists, mind healers, scientists, hypnotists or simply outstanding individuals in any sphere of life perhaps stumbled on the discovery of vital energy without knowing its nature. However, the vital energy can be used consciously. A common example in the Western world are pregnant women who are taught certain types of breathing exercises for less painful childbirth.

The correct habit of breathing, along with a natural diet, can regenerate people for whom the modern diseases of civilized man, such as blood pressure, heart diseases, asthma, etc. would be only medical names in the dictionary. In addition to the physical benefits derived through breathing, use of correct breathing can also increase will power, self-control, power of concentration, moral qualities, and even spiritual evolution.

This chapter is intended to promote awareness about proper breathing. By understanding and following the breathing exercises, one can continually monitor and improve one's health, vitality, and emotions.

Parts of the Body Involved in Breathing

Lungs Structure and Function: As most of us may already know, the lungs are spongy and porous and their tissues are very elastic. They contain innumerable air sacs. The right lung consists of three lobes and the left one two lobes (Fig. 7.1). When we breathe, we draw in air through the nose (and sometimes mouth); after it has passed through the nose and the pharynx and the larynx, it passes into the trachea or windpipe, which in turn is subdivided into innumerable smaller tubes called bronchioles. The bronchioles terminate in minute subdivisions in the small air sacs called alveoli, whose number is approximately 600 million. Each of these air sacs or alveoli holds a portion of the inhaled air, from which the oxygen penetrates through the walls of the pulmonary capillaries. Then the blood takes up oxygen and releases carbon dioxide generated from the waste products that have been gathered up by the blood from all parts of the system. Owing to the contact of the blood, the air sacs are now drained of the pure oxygen and in turn they are filled with carbon dioxide from the blood. The efficiency of gaseous exchange is facilitated by the large surface area of the lungs. The volume of the lungs of an average-sized adult varies from four to six liters, or about the amount of air contained in a basketball. If lung tissue is spread out like a carpet it would cover half a tennis court, or about 35 times the surface area of a person. At any one time there is about one pint of blood in the fine network of blood vessels surrounding the lung tissue. The overall arrangement of lung tissue and blood vessels provides a tremendous interface for the aeration of blood with the environment. How air is brought into the lungs (inhalation) and squeezed out of the lungs (exhalation) is described in the next section. The control over inhalation and exhalation is important to increase the amount of oxygen intake providing energy.

Mechanics of Breathing: Before learning breathing exercises, it is important to understand the mechanical arrangements whereby respiratory movements are affected. The trunk is divided into two portions, the (upper) thoracic cavity and (lower) abdominal cavity (see Fig. 7.1). These cavities are separated by the muscular partition known as the diaphragm that plays an important role in respiration. The elastic movement of the lungs and the activities of the side and bottom of the thoracic cavity carry on the process of respiration. The thoracic cavity, which holds the lungs and heart, is bounded by the spinal column, the ribs, and the breast bone.

In the process of inhalation, the ribs are moved by the intercostal muscles and the diaphragm descends (as much as four inches) towards the abdominal cavity. The movement of the ribs and the intercostal muscles and the pull of the diaphragm downward expand the two elastic lungs. When the lungs are expanded a vacuum is created and the air from outside rushes in through the nose and mouth. The degree of lung filling depends on the magnitude of movements of the diaphragm and the respiratory muscles. The practice of complete breathing, as discussed later, involves the proper control of the diaphragm and the respiratory muscles, which will bring the maximum degree of lung expansion in order to absorb the greatest amount of oxygen from the air. The exhalation or breathing out occurs mainly as a result of returning the diaphragm upward by the relaxation of the respiratory muscles.

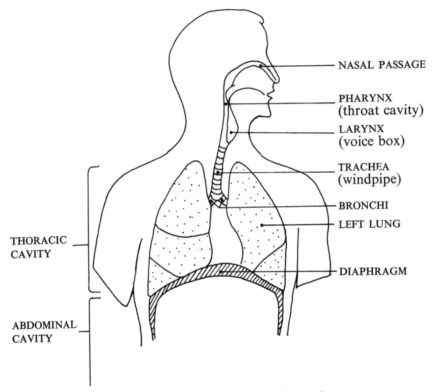

Fig. 7.1. Diagrammatic representation of the respiratory system.

Types of Breathing

Breathing practices can be divided into 3 types, which are based on the involvement of diaphragm and respiratory muscles. These differ in bringing the amount of air into the lungs and the efforts involved. After understanding these 3 types of breathing, we will discuss the fourth type called *complete breathing* or *yogic breathing* or *total breathing*, which should be adopted for improving vigor and vitality.

1. *Deep Breathing (or Low Breathing):* You may have been suggested to take a deep breath at a time of nervousness such as going for an interview or speaking in front of an audience for the first time. When you take a deep breath, you breathe all the way to your stomach, and you are practicing deep or low breathing. The lungs are employed far more extensively in low breathing than in the other two kinds. However, they are still not completely filled with vital and necessary oxygen as you will realize later during complete breathing.

In deep breathing, the diaphragm is descended without raising the chest and shoulders. When the diaphragm contracts and its dome-shaped center becomes flattened, it thereby pushes the abdominal contents and makes the abdomen bulge out. Here the ribs and the intercostal muscles are at rest. By watching the abdominal movements, you can easily discover that on inspiration, as the dome-shaped diaphragm flattens, the abdomen bulges out, and the cubic capacity of the chest increases and the air rushes in. As the diaphragm returns to its original position, the abdomen moves in and air is forced our of the lungs.

2. *Chest Breathing* (*or Mid Breathing*):   In this type the chest is expanded without involving the diaphragm. Here the intercostal muscles of the rib expand the lungs partially and the diaphragm is in neutral position. The breathing is done absolutely through the actions of the respiratory muscles connected with the ribs. Chest breathing commonly occurs during physical work and exercise. The stomach muscles during these activities become tense, and thus interfere with descending of the diaphragm.

3. *High Breathing:*   Here the inspiration, involves raising the shoulders and collarbone while the abdomen is contracted. Neither the diaphragm nor intercostal muscles are used. Most of us, especially those in sedentary occupations, are high breathers. Whenever we sit or lean over the desk to work, the chest and stomach tend to collapse, thus preventing the complete inflation of the entire lung area. The high breather is characterized by a quick and shallow breathing pattern necessary to provide sufficient oxygen.

To find out the difference for yourself among the three types of breathing, count the number of seconds you take to fill the lungs. You will note down the "Deep or Low Breathing" brings in more air to the lungs with less effort than the other two types of breathing. But the "Chest or Mid Breathing" is better than "High Breathing." The third "High Breathing" is the worst of all breathings, where shoulders and collarbones are raised and the abdomen is contracted while inhaling. The high breathers use the most energy to get very little air. Many diseases of the vocal organs and the respiratory system are noted in those who use this method of breathing. The common disease of asthma, noted more often in people with "High Breathing" habit, has been reported to be corrected by changing the breathing habits according to a complete breathing practice along with proper diet.

As noted above, the best breathing among the three types is "Deep Breathing" or "Low Breathing," where the diaphragm plays the major role. When the diaphragm is brought to use in "Deep (or Low) Breathing," it presses upon the abdominal organs and forces out the abdomen. Naturally in this type of breathing the lungs are given more space and freer play than in the other two types.

Though the deep or low abdominal breathing involving the diaphragm is the best, yet it is not itself a complete breathing exercise. The reason is that any one of these breathing methods fills only a portion of the lungs—the low breathing the lower and middle parts, chest breathing the middle and a portion of the upper regions, and the high breathing the upper portion of the lungs.

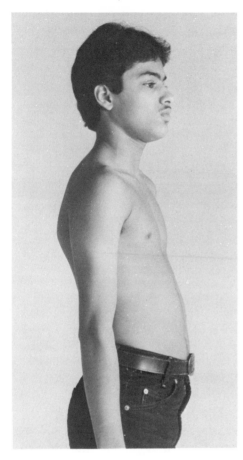 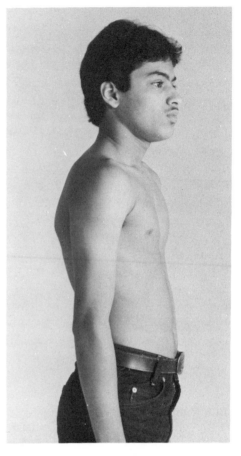

Step 1. Relax your stomach and allow it to bulge out as you fill the lower lungs with air.

Step 2. Expand your ribs and let the breath fill your mid-section.

Fig. 7.2. Stepwise illustrations of Complete Breathing.

4. *Complete Breathing or Yogic Breathing or Total Breathing:* The practice of complete breathing involves the use of all three methods of breathing simultaneously, starting with low breathing, continuing the chest breathing, and finally finishing with high breathing. During this type of inhalation process, the whole respiratory system comes into play and no portion of the lungs is left unfilled with fresh air.

To practice the use of the whole respiratory system in complete breathing, try the following steps (as illustrated in Fig. 7.2) either in an easy standing position or in a sitting position such as one of the meditative poses or in a chair. (1) Inhale slowly using the diaphragm as in deep breathing. Aim the breath below the stomach and notice the stomach bulging out. This will fill the lower part of the lungs with air. (2) Continue to breathe and fill the mid-section by expanding the rib section outward to the sides as in chest breathing. (3) Finally, fill the uppermost

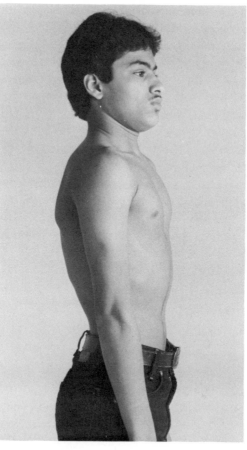

Step 3. While lifting up the chest area, continue the breath so that it fills the upper chest and lungs.

part of the lungs by lifting up the chest area as in high breathing. The entire process of inhalation should be completed in about four seconds. Eventually with practice you can increase the time of inhalation, and adjust retention and exhalation time in proper proportion as discussed in the next section. (4) Try to retain for eight seconds. The longer time gives the lungs a good chance to use and absorb all the oxygen. (5) Begin exhalation by gently contracting the lower stomach. This will push out the air in the lowest part of the lungs. As the lower lungs empty themselves of their air, the rib section will slowly deflate, followed by the upper chest. The exhalation should be done slowly in about twice the time of inhalation so that the maximum amount of old foul air is squeezed out. Pause for a few seconds before beginning the next inhalation.

Ratio of Inhalation, Retention and Exhalation in Complete Breathing

In complete breathing the greatest attention is given to the process of exhalation; the time ratio between inhalation and exhalation is 1:2. If the inhaltion is one second, the exhalation will be two seconds. The reason for making the exhalation

longer than inhalation is to get maximum control over the lungs so that old foul
air sacs can be squeezed out. As long as the air sacs are filled with old air, no
amount of strength applied in inhalation can bring fresh air from the atmosphere.
In ordinary breathing we squeeze out a very little volume of air from the upper
part of the lungs, leaving the lower part almost inactive. Some people use only the
base of the lungs for breathing, leaving the upper portion idle. As we learn the
complete use of lungs, the more air is squeezed out, and consequently the more
fresh air rushes into the lungs from the atmosphere, as there cannot be any
vacuum in the air sacs. Therefore, the first step of complete breathing is to keep
the inhalation and exhalation ratio of 1 : 2, starting with four seconds of inhalation
and eight seconds of exhalation. Then slowly increase the time of both inhalation
and exhalation, maintaining the ratio of 1 : 2.

After properly establishing the inhalation and exhalation, the next step is to
retain the breath proportionately. The ratio between inhalation and retention is
1 : 4. Since the retention is four times inhalation, and exhalation is always twice
inhalation, therefore the ratio between inhalation, retention and exhalation is
1 : 4 : 2. The minimum schedule is to start with four seconds of inhalation with
corresponding sixteen seconds of retention and eight seconds of exhalation.

Breathing Exercises

All the breathing exercises should utilize low, mid, and high breathing as described
in complete breathing in the section on types of breathing. The important starting
exercise is the alternate breathing exercise. The reason for doing alternate breathing
is that the breath alternates between two nostrils. You can easily find out for yourself by placing your palm near the nostrils. One of the nostrils is always partially
blocked, and the flow of air in and out of the lungs is mainly through only one of
the nostrils. If a person is in normal health, and has perfected breathing, the
breath will alternate approximately every hour and fifty minutes. In the majority of
people this change of the breath from one nostril to the other, however, varies due
to such conditions as unnatural living habits, wrong diet, diseases, and the lack
of proper exercises.

According to yogic philosophy, if the air flow in right nostril is more active, the
metabolic activity of the body is abnormally high, and there will be mental and
nervous disturbances. When the left nostril is more active, the metabolic activity
of the body becomes low, thus producing suspended mental activity.Thus, in Yoga,
alternate breathing exercises are mainly for the purpose of maintaining equilibrium.

Single Nostril Breathing Exercise: Sit in any one of the meditative poses, such
as the lotus or adept's or easy pose (see Chapter 8), keeping the spine, neck, and
head in a straight line. Close the right nostril with your thumb or fore-finger
(see Fig. 7.3). Inhale slowly through the left nostril, counting five. Exhale through
the same nostril counting ten to keep the proportion of inhalation to exhalation

at 1:2. Repeat this exercise fifteen to twenty rounds through the left nostril, keeping the proportion at five seconds inhalation and ten seconds exhalation. Now close the left nostril, and inhale through the right nostril counting five. Exhale through the same nostril counting ten to keep the proportion of inhalation to exhalation at 1:2. Repeat this exercise fifteen to twenty rounds as for the left nostril.

Do not make any sound during inhalation. Apply the basic rules of low, mid, and high breathing during inhalation. During exhalation, try to expel as much as possible of the foul air from the lungs.

Practice this Single Nostril Breathing Exercise for fifteen days to a month and slowly increase the proportion to six seconds inhalation and twelve seconds exhalation. Do not try the higher proportion until you are able to do the lower proportion very easily.

In the Single Nostril Breathing Exercise there is no retention or holding of the breath. The purpose of inhaling and exhaling through one nostril is to establish the use of each nostril for the purpose of maintaining an equilibrium between breath alternation. Unless one is able to do low, mid, and high breathing perfectly and automatically, he should not attempt advanced breathing exercises.

Alternate Breathing Exercise: A month of practicing Single Nostril Breathing Exercise is sufficient. Now you need not practice Single Nostril Breathing, and can start the Alternate Breathing Exercise. As illustrated in Figure 7.3, close the right nostril with your right thumb and inhale through the left nostril (Fig. 7.3, Step 1). Now close the left nostril immediately with your right fore-finger (Fig. 7.3, Step 2). Remove your thumb from the right nostril and exhale through the right nostril. This is a half round.

Now without pausing, inhale through the right nostril. Close the right nostril with your right thumb and exhale through the left. This makes one full round.

The proportion of inhalation to exhalation is 1:2 or six seconds inhalation and twelve seconds exhalation. The same general rules for the Single Nostril Breathing Exercise apply for Alternate Breathing Exercise as well. Do fifteen to twenty rounds.

You should practice this exercise two to three months and finally increasing to eight and sixteen seconds inhalation and exhalation. Within this period you should see tremendous changes taking place in your body and mind. The breathing will become perfect, especially the movement of the diaphragm; and the body becomes very light and the eyes shine.

Full Alternate Breathing Exercise: In this exercise we include retention or holding of the breath. This is the only difference between the Alternate Breathing and the Full Alternate Breathing Exercise.

The correct ratio between inhalation and retention is 1:4, but beginners are advised to follow a 1:2 ratio for a few months before taking up the 1:4 ratio. The minimum starting proportion is four seconds inhalation, eight seconds retention, and eight seconds exhalation. After a month, increase to 5:10:10 and gradually to 8:16:16.

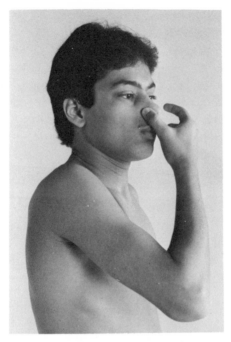 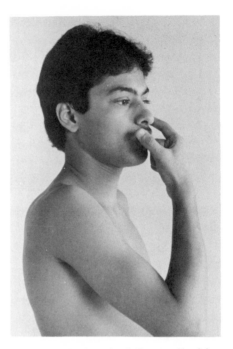

Step 1. Keeping right nostril closed
with a thumb, inhale through
the left nostril.

Step 2. Closing the left nostril with
fore finger, release the thumb
and exhale through the right
nostril.

Fig. 7.3. Stepwise illustrations of Alternate Breathing Exercise.

Inhale the air through the left nostril while counting four. Retain the air counting eight. Exhale through the right nostril while counting eight. Now without
stopping, inhale through right nostril, retain the breath, and exhale through the
left nostril—all in the same 4:8:8 proportion. This is one full round. Practice
fifteen to twenty rounds daily.

When you are able to do 8:16:16 comfortably, change the ratio to 1:4:2. Start
with four seconds inhalation, sixteen seconds retention, and eight seconds exhalation. Gradually work up to 8:32:16. It should take eight to twelve months of
practice to reach this timing. Do not try to rush it.

When done properly, certain signs are visible during the exercise period. In
the first stage, the body perspires. In the second stage a tremor is felt throughout
the body, making one feel fresh and energetic.

Abdominal or Diaphragmatic Breathing Exercise: One should start this exercise
only after practicing the Alternate Breathing Exercise for one or two months
because many people need quite a time to get the diaphragm to move properly
during breathing. The vast majority tend to breathe incorrectly by contracting the
abdominal muscles and raising the shoulders while inhaling, which is in direct
contrast to correct breathing. Therefore, until the diaphragm takes the natural
movement, one should not practice abdominal breathing.

To practice abdominal breathing, it is advisable to use the lotus position if possible. This position includes the foot lock, which holds a person in place throughout the exercise.

In this exercise, exhalation plays a prominent part. Inhalation is mild, slow, and longer than exhalation. In the other breathing exercises mentioned above, exhalation is longer than inhalation.

In the Abdominal Breathing Exercise, inhalation and exhalation are performed by the abdominal muscles and the diaphragm. Inhalation and exhalation are performed in quick succession by a sudden and vigorous intake of the abdominal muscles, followed by relaxation of the abdominal muscles. Exhalation takes about one-fourth the time of inhalation. Here exhalation is quick, strong, and short, while inhalation is passive, slow, and longer. Passive inhalation and a sudden expulsion of breath follow continuously, one after the other, until a round is completed. In the beginning, a round should have fifteen to twenty expulsions. You can add the expulsions each week until you reach one hundred twenty expulsions in each round. Between rounds, take a few normal breaths while resting. According to the individual condition, increase the number of rounds without overdoing it. While practicing Abdominal Breathing your attention should be concentrated on the abdominal muscles.

This exercise cleans the respiratory system and the nasal passages and removes spasms in bronchial tubes. Consequently, asthma is relieved and may even be cured in the course of time. The apices of the lungs get proper oxygenation, carbon dioxide is eliminated, and oxygen is absorbed into the system. This is the best exercise to increase oxygen in the system.

Surya Bedha Breathing Exercise: To practice this exercise, sit in any meditative pose such as the adept's pose (*Sidhasan*). Keep the left nostril closed and without making any sound inhale as long as you can through the right nostril. Then close the right nostril with your right thumb and retain the breath by firmly pressing the chin against the chest (the chin lock).

Increase the retention gradually. Then exhale very slowly without making any sound through the left nostril by closing the right nostril. In this breathing exercise, inhalation is always through the right nostril. Start with ten rounds and gradually increase to forty rounds.

The proper practice of this breathing exercise can cure pulmonary, cardiac, and dropsical disease. It also cleanses the frontal sinuses and preserves the physical health.

Applications of Breathing in Daily Activities

Unlike food, air is breathed every second. It is the oxygen we breathe that fuels the working of our cells, and provides the basic life force that keeps us going. Biologically, oxygen is required for the body's metabolism, which provides energy for physical and mental activity, as well as for the on going involuntary functioning of the body. The breathing practices in the following pages can be used to recharge the body and can thus replace such harmful stimulants as coffee and smoking. It is hoped that you will like at least some of the exercises, which suits the most to your needs.

Breathing for Energy at Work:

1. Sit comfortably in a chair and place your hands on your thighs.
2. Form your lips into an "O" and relax your tongue so that it does not block the passage of air. Now suck in air through the mouth, filling first the lower part of the lungs, then the rib area and finally the upper chest. This should all be done in one strong inhalation. Your breath should sound like a gust of wind. Your rib cage should be fully expanded and your posture fully erect.
3. Hold the breath for four seconds.
4. Exhale by forcefully blowing the breath out through the open mouth.
5. Repeat this sucking inhalation two more times.
6. On the last exhalation, gently blow the air out as if cooling a spoon of soup.
7. Repeat three times.

The energizing breath can be used at any time of the day when you feel the need for a quick pick up. After three repetitions, the body will once again feel alert.

Alternate Breathing for Vitalization:

1. Sit comfortably in a chair and rest your left hand on a thigh.
2. Close the right nostril with your right thumb.
3. Now slowly inhale the complete breath through the left nostril for ten counts.
4. With the right fore-finger close the left nostril and hold the breath for ten counts.
5. To exhale, release only the thumb and slowly exhale through the right nostril for ten counts.
6. Pause for two counts.
7. Keeping the right nostril open, slowly inhale the total breath for ten counts.
8. Now, close the right nostril with the thumb and hold the breath for ten counts.
9. Exhale through the left nostril for ten counts by releasing the fore-finger only.
10. Pause for two counts. Continue the breath by alternating the nostrils until you have inhaled ten times through each side.

After finishing the exercise, you will feel calm waves of energy flowing through your entire body. The first few times you practice the breath you may feel slightly dizzy or light-headed. This is because your body is not accustomed to a wave of clean energy.

Breathing and Stretching for Stimulation:
- a. 1. Standing with your feet apart, inhale a complete breath and hold.
  2. Place your hands on your hips and bend backward as far as possible. Notice the wonderful stretching and loosening you feel along the spine. As you bend backward, exhale fully.
  3. Remain in this position for as long as possible without strain.
  4. Slowly return to the standing position. As you do so breathe in the complete breath.
  5. Repeat three times.
- b. 1. Stand erect with your hands at your sides.
  2. Begin to inhale the complete breath. As you inhale slowly, begin to raise your arms in front of you and up over your head.
  3. Hold the breath and stretch as much as possible.
  4. Slowly bring your arms down to your sides, and exhale through your nose.
  5. Repeat the entire exercise three times.

Breathing and Bending:
1. Stand with hands on hips and feet apart.
2. Inhale the complete breath.
3. Without bending the knees, bend forward from the waist, keeping your trunk straight. As you bend forward, exhale. (See "Warm-up Exercise" in Chapter 8.)
4. As you come back up, inhale a lung-full of air.
5. Pause momentarily and again bend forward and exhale.
6. Continue the exercise for fifteen counts.

Breathing for Joggers:
1. To inhale, push the stomach out and let the air rush in to fill the rib-cage area and finally the upper chest. Be sure to expand your rib cage out as far as possible to allow in a good supply of air.
2. To exhale, slightly contract the stomach and then let the air release itself progressively from the mid area and then the chest areas.
3. Continue breathing in this fashion as you jog.

To prevent cramping as well as to establish a steady rhythm to sustain you during the jogging, each inhalation and exhalation should be done slowly to the count of ten. Keeping the count mentally, focuses the attention on a steady rhythm and keeps your mind off the feelings of fatigue or anxiety.

Breathing to Relax:
1. Gently inhale following the low, mid and high technique of complete breath.
2. Hold the breath for three seconds.
3. Clench your teeth and open your lips. Force the air out between the teeth. You will be making a hissing sound like a tea kettle.

4. Repeat four times. You can vary the intensity of the exhalation and the hissing.

Breathing to Replace Smoking:

1. Forcefully inhale a complete breath. Breathe in as deeply as possible.
2. Hold the breath for two seconds.
3. Tilt your head slightly back and exhale through your mouth with great force. As you exhale, shape your lips into a tiny "O" so that the air has to be forced out during the exhalation. Pull in your stomach with the exhalation so that the air is really forced out.
4. After repeating this breath three or four times, finish off with a regular complete breath.
5. After the initial cigarette craving has left, you may want to repeat this exercise, only a bit more gently. Often people find themselves yawning briefly after this exercise, as the body accommodates itself to a new supply of fresh oxygen.

Breathing for Stress and Emotions:

a. 1. Standing, spread your legs as far apart as possible.
    2. Exhale and bend forward from the waist, letting your arms between your legs. Try to bring your head down to knee level.
    3. Start your inhalation with your head lowered at knee level.
    4. Bring your arms slowly up over your head as you breathe in the complete breath.
    5. Bend backward, retaining the breath, and repeat the exhalation.
    6. Repeat the exercise five times.

Lowering the head in this exercise helps to improve the blood supply that carries oxygen to the brain. Normally the blood has to work harder to make its oxygen delivery to parts of the body above the heart. A poor oxygen supply to the brain is indicated by fatigue, irritability, and moodiness.

b. 1. Using the fingertips of your left hand, rub the palm of your right hand in a clockwise direction as if you were rubbing a smooth stone. Do this twenty times. Then turn the right hand over and rub the back of the hand for twenty times.
    2. Reverse hands and rub the palm of the left hand with your right hand twenty times. Again, turn the hand over and rub its back twenty times.
    3. Now place the tips of your fingers gently over your closed eyelids, slightly pressing in. Your palms should cup your cheeks.
    4. Inhale the complete breath.
    5. Retain for ten counts.
    6. Exhale.
    7. Repeat the entire exercise two more times.

By rubbing the hands you stimulate the circulation of your hands, creating a slight warmth or tingling sensation. This is a soothing as well as a revitalizing energy that stills the mind for clearer thought.

Breathing for Sleep:

- a. 1. Lying flat on your back with your hands by your sides, close your eyes. Slowly begin to inhale the complete breath through your nose. As you inhale, begin to raise your arms in an arc up and over your head.
  2. Continue to inhale very slowly for the count of ten or until your arms reach back at the bed and are stretched out over your head.
  3. Hold the breath for ten counts.
  4. As you exhale to a count of ten, slowly return your arms in the arc until they are resting alongside your body.
  5. Repeat the exercise ten times.
  6. Go to sleep.

With each inhalation you will begin to fall deeper and deeper into an almost dreamlike state. By lifting your arms up and over your head as you breathe you give your lungs the chance to expand fully and take in a larger supply of oxygen. This increased oxygen is invaluable for quieting nerves and producing a deep and restful sleep.

The above exercise not only solves the difficulties of falling asleep but also prepares the body for a deeper and richer sleep. If at first you cannot fulfill the count of ten, breathe in five, hold five and release five. Then gradually work your way up to ten.

- b. 1. Lying flat on your back in a relaxed state, inhale slowly through both nostrils in a steady but controlled stream.
  2. As soon as you have inhaled the maximum amount of air possible without straining, immediately let the breath exhale by itself. Do not hold the breath or pause between inhalations.
  3. When you have just finished exhaling, begin another inhalation, again without pausing.
  4. Slowly repeat this exercise ten times.
  5. Progressively take longer and longer with each inhalation and exhalation. At the end of the exercise, you will be drifting off to sleep.

- c. If you find yourself occasionally waking in the middle of the night after a few hours of sleep, try the following steps.
  1. Lying flat on your back in bed, close the right nostril with the right thumb.
  2. Slowly inhale through the left nostril for ten counts. As you inhale, aim the breath for the spot in the center of your forehead (*Ajna Chakra*, representing mind's eye between two eyebrows).
  3. Hold the breath for ten counts.
  4. Still holding the right nostril closed, exhale for ten counts.
  5. After pausing for five counts, close the left nostril with the middle finger.

6. Slowly inhale for ten counts, again aiming for that spot in the middle of the forehead.
7. Hold for a count of ten.
8. Still holding the left nostril closed, exhale for ten counts. Repeat the above steps ten times, after which you should quickly be on the way back to sleep. When practicing the above steps watch your inhalations to make sure that they are silent. If they whistle at all, inhale at a slower, more even pace. The same rule applies to exhalations.

One of the most important keys to achieving a thorough night's rest is the ability to relax while going to sleep. If you let problems of the day intrude into your mind just before you retire, chances are your sleep will be uneven and usually disturbed. Therefore, the relaxation of mind for sleep as described in Chapter 2 is an integral part of sleep program.

A Word of Caution

The breathing exercises mentioned above are safe and effective in stimulating body metabolism. With proper practice they should help one to feel vigor and vitality in daily activities. Advanced yogic breathing and the use of locks for awakening the Serpent Power (*Kundalini Shakti*) should be tried only under the guidance of an expert yoga teacher (Guru); these in my opinion are not required by an average person to maintain good health and vitality.

In the advanced yogic practices, the yogis augment the postures (*asanas*) and breathing practices (*pranayama*) by muscular locks or *bandhas*. The tensing of certain inner muscles, stimulate the three vital plexuses—in the throat, abdomen, and base of the spine. These contractions increase muscular tone and coordination and galvanize the whole nervous system. They produce an electrical current or force called *Kundalini Shakti* (serpent power). *Kundalini Shakti* is a spiritual force that is pictured as lying coiled like a serpent at the base of the spine while in its dormant stage. It can be raised by violent breathing practices and other Hatha Yoga methods. It can also be aroused through other methods, such as through devotion and love for God, through intense meditation on the *Kundalini*, and through the power of the analytical will of the *Gyana* Yoga. In most people, *Kundalini* is suggested to ascend or descend between the first three of seven *chakras* or wheels or centers that represent specific areas of the body along the spinal cord (the lowest at the base of the spine and highest at the crown of the head). Only in evolved spirituals, it rises to the highest of seven *chakras* (*Sahasrara*). The yogis devote their life to the practice of such advanced techniques for controlling psychological and physiological forces. These practices often do not suit the life style of an average person. Moreover, any attempt to awaken the *Kundalini Shakti* without long and elaborate preparations without the necessary preconditions and lacking the guidance of a *Guru* can lead to serious mental and physical problems.

Chapter 8

Walking and Yogic Exercises for Health

Clearly, most people accept the proposition that exercise improves strength and stamina, and provides an overall sense of well-being. Yet strenuous exercises are too tiring and even risky for individuals of older age and those with diseased conditions. Overexercising can be dangerous even for a healthy person. For example, strenuous exericises resulting in excessive loss of body fat in young healthy women upset the hormonal balance, and result in irregular or no menstruation; a situation that requires medical treatment. Walking and yogic exercises, on the other hand, are not only suitable for people of all ages and physique but keep older people young and cure many stressrelated diseases.

The Miracle of Walking

Whatever ails you, one of the best cures is a good, brisk walk. It may not cure everything, you understand, but walking helps circulation by speeding blood to the heart; it soothes nervous tension, relieves anxiety, and eases frustration. The rewards of walking for most people equal those of glamorous sports such as swimming, tennis, skiing and scuba diving. Walking also maintains the weight at a proper level, regulates the appetite, keeps the bones from weakening, improves the looks and burns off fat. Most of all, walking gives us the opportunity to think and relax as we give our body a chance to unwind. Walking after dinner helps to get a good sleep, especially for sedentary workers.

When walking increases the blood's oxygen-carrying capacity, more oxygen is supplied faster and more efficiently. The result of this is faster recovery from illness and accidents. Walking lowers the blood pressure and helps prevent gout by lowering uric acid level. It makes arteries more elastic and the whole body more flexible and strong.

When combined with a natural diet, walking constitutes the best possible defense against degenerative aging conditions. Atherosclerosis and all of its nasty results respond best to the combination of diet and exercise. Of course, of the two, diet is the most important. Only diet, for example, can effectively reduce cholesterol levels.

Breathing during the Walk: Correct breathing adds to stamina and endurance, especially when we are covering miles of ground as, for example, during hiking. The complete breath as discussed in the previous chapter is the best all-around breath to insure proper oxygenation of the body. Start with low breathing and continue with mid and high breathing to utilize the lungs at their full capacity. The breathing rate, in general, should be comfortable, never too quick or too slow. An easy check of proper breathing during a walk is that your rate of breathing should never interfere with your ability to carry on a conversation. An easy natural rhythm of movement and posture is crucial. The head should be floating nicely on the neck, not held with rigidity or cramped. The spine should be naturally erect but not to the point of strain. This will help you breathe in an unrestrained manner.

Starting out the Walk: One who has not walked for a long while should start slowly. Walk the distance you feel comfortable with. After about three days, increase the distance by 10 percent. After about a week increase that distance by another 10 percent. Following this strategy, the walking distance will be doubled in about 5 weeks, which is a safe and effective way to increase your distance.

The speed at which you walk is less important than the distance. Increase your walking speed only after you have had about five weeks of conditioning. If you are walking four or five miles at a time, and can maintain a brisk pace, you may be ready for jogging, if you choose.

It is important not to walk or jog faster than you should. To check this, stop and rest after walking or jogging for a full minute. Now count your pulse rate for a minute.* When you are really in shape, your pulse rate per minute should be about 100, even if you have been exercising strenuously. If your pulse exceeds 130, slow down until your body is ready for increasing the distance or speed.

Keeping up the Walk: As far back as I can recall, walking after dinner has been one of my regular habits—similar to eating and sleeping—and this has been my most relaxing and stress-relieving experience. The deep breath of fresh air and thinking about whatever you like provides such a joy that your are likely to continue the walk. However, the following points should be helpful in keeping up the walking until it is incorporated as a habit in your life.

1. The main secret in maintaining a daily walk or other exercise is to establish a top priority. The excuse of not being able to find the time is a cop-out. We find time to sleep because it is mandatory. So is walking or other exercise. Arrange a simple schedule that works well for you. Walk every morning before work or during lunch or in the evening. You have to tell yourself

---

* Pulse is usually counted at the wrist. A little below the base of the thumb, just inside the point where a projection of the wristbone can be felt on the thumb side, an artery runs under the skin of the inner surface of the wrist. Place your fingertips (not thumb) on this part of the wrist. Press just hard enough for pulsations to be felt. Count either for 30 seconds and multiply by two or count for a full minute. Average adult has a pulse rate of 70 to 72 per minute, but this can vary a little in either direction and still be normal. Activity, excitement, and illness can cause changes in the pulse rate. The pulse can also be taken in areas other than a wrist where an artery crosses bone near the skin surface—for instance, at the temples, or between the ankle bone and heel on the inner side of the foot.

that you are the most important person, and that nothing is more important than your life and your walking.

2. The company of a good friend or a relative can be helpful to keep up with the walking schedule.

3. When driving to work, park half a mile away from work; whenever you travel a short distance, walk instead of taking a car or bus. For variety, alternate between riding a bicycle and walking, but remember that walking is a far better exercise.

4. If you like to keep a dog, it will get you out walking.

5. Weather can be the most common excuse for many of us, but we can always figure out a way of getting in our daily walk, no matter what kind of weather prevails. Find any large space to walk in a department store, shopping mall, building concourse, or your own basement. Use the stairs insted of the elevator.

Yogic Exercises for Daily Practice at Home

The word Yoga means union, and it is taken literally to mean union of a mind with a healthy body so that the two can work together. Yoga is not really a simple set of exercises. It aspires to develop body, mind, and spirit, all three of which according to yogic philosophy must be fully developed before we can realize our full potential. The yoga way of life has been practiced for over 6,000 years. Although yoga is generally associated with two populous religions of the East, Hinduism and Buddhism, it is not a prerequisite for either religion; and Yoga philosophy does not quarrel with any religion or faith. Yoga is now practiced by people, irrespective of religion and it has been absorbed in the West as much as in the East.

To sum up the implications of yoga to a Westerner, we can cite a short verse from the words of Guru Nanak, the founder of the Sikh religion.

> The world is an ocean, and difficult to cross,
> How shall man traverse it?
> As a lotus in the water remaineth dry,
> As also a water fowl in the stream—
> So by meditating on the word,
> Shalt thou be unaffected by the world.

The four broad forms of yoga include (1) *Karma Yoga* (path of action) (2) *Bhakti Yoga* (path of devotion) (3) *Gyan Yoga* (path of knowledge) (4) *Raja Yoga* (the science of mental control). Again, Raja Yoga has been divided into three more subdivisions known as *Mantra Yoga, Kundalini Yoga* and *Hatha Yoga* which are various modes of practice. The name Hatha Yoga is perhaps most familiar to us and can be divided as follows:

1. Purification of the body (*Yama*).

2. Practice of postures (*Asanas*) or yogic exercises.

3. Practice of Mudras and Bandhas which produce electrical current or force called Serpent Power (*Kundalini Shakti*).
4. Control of vital breath through yogic breathing (*Pranayama*).
5. Stilling of the mind and its modifications by cutting off the sense perception (*Prathyahara*).
6. Progression in mental control or concentration (*Dharana*).
7. Meditation on various nerve centers, which makes the mind steady (*Dhyana*).
8. The highest superconscious state, when the little ego 'I' merges with the supreme Ego or God.

The adoption of a full yogic life style is a life-time devotion that is not practical for most of us. To make the best of it while doing our worldly duties, postures or yogic exercises are an important addition to our daily routine for training of the physical body and mind.

The exercises contained here can be practiced with safety and are ideal for everyone wishing to attain a perfect health. The yogic exercises differ from other physical exercises in that, due to the slow movements of various joints, blood vessels are pulled and stretched and the blood is equally distributed to every part of the body. The stretched muscles and ligaments during the yogic practice are immediately relaxed, carrying more energy to the muscle fibers. Deep breathing with mild retention during the practice allows for more oxygen absorption. Yogic exercises also keep the proper curvature of the spine and increase its flexibility by stretching the anterior and posterior longitudinal ligaments. The ligaments (which connect bone and other structures) in an average individual become stiff and many people cannot touch the floor, even at the age of twenty. The stiffening of backbone, a common problem related to age, can be avoided by daily practice of yogic postures. Yoga has also been shown to help stress-related problems such as high blood pressure.

There are 840,000 poses according to the *Yoga Shastras*, of which only important ones are given here. If one does not have time to practice all of the exercises and needs to make a selection, it must be remembered that the principal rule in the performance of any exercise is that it is to be countered with a performance of its direct opposite. For example, if a forward bending exercise is selected, it is imperative that a backward bending exercise is performed to offset it.

The exercises in the following pages are laid out in an orderly sequence. These can be alternated for the sake of variety and over-all body coverage as one progresses.

Many of these exercises may seem difficult to a number of beginners. However, contrary to what many people believe, yoga is not a regime of painful body contortions. These postures are the exercises that can eventually be performed (at least, many of them) by individuals of various ages and body build. Since the performance of these exercises is an ultimate goal, the beginners are not given any separate set of exercises. They can, however, start with doing a part of the posture, for example, bending halfway, and then gradually working towards a complete posture, as body flexibility increases. Whatever part of the posture one can perform without hurting is useful. Do not rush yourself. When a posture causes discomfort, it is time to stop it. Although postures do, in fact, aim to increase the mobility and suppleness of the body, the most important part of yoga is that it is a way to deep mental relaxation.

Making sure not to eat beforehand (wait three hours after meals), you should start yoga postures (asanas) by relaxing and recharging the body along with readjusting the psyche. As described later for the relaxation posture, this is performed while lying on the back with arms along sides, palms up, quieting yourself and keeping your body loose. After closing the eyes, relax the whole body from toes to head, breathing in slowly and deeply from the diaphragm. Relazation should be practiced two to three minutes or longer if required; it is useful to practice after each major exercise or sequence of positions in order to keep yourself refreshed.

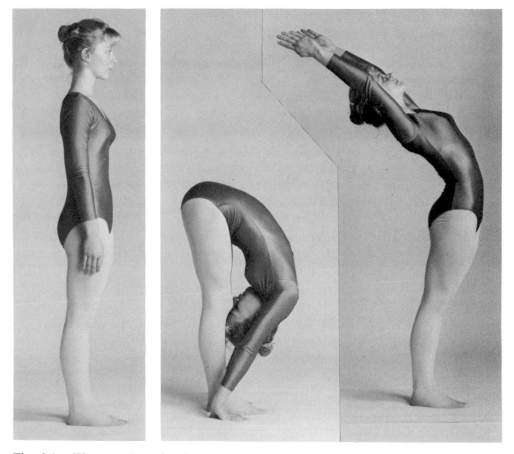

Fig. 8.1. Warm-up Stretches (*Soorya Namaskar*)
Position 1

Fig. 8.3. Warm-up Stretches
(*Soorya Namaskar*)
Position 3

Fig. 8.2. Warm-up Stretches (*Soorya Namaskar*)
Position 2

Warm-up: These exercises loosen and tone muscles in the back, shoulders and legs and prepares the body for the postures (asanas) to follow.

Stand erect with arms at sides (Position 1). Exhale and bend forward; if possible, touch your head with your knees, resting your hands on the floor (Position 2). Keep the knees straight. It will probably be some time before many of us can do this, depending upon our bone structure and body condition. In any case, bend as far as possible without hurting yourself and then slowly move back to a full standing posture.

Inhaling, stretch the spine, head and arms forward and then up to the ceiling and finally backward (Position 3). Exhale, as you lower the arms to the sides, and relax. Perform the above steps slowly and repeat four times. You should feel a relaxing sensation while lowering the arms.

Forward Bending Exercises: These exercises flatten the stomach, slim the waist, firm the thighs, loosen the spine, tone the body, aid the digestion, and eliminate constipation.

Plough Pose (Halasana): Lie flat on your back with arms at your sides and palms on the floor. Slowly raise legs and hips off the floor in a continuous movement. Tilt your legs over your head until the toes touch the floor, beyond the head. Press the chin against the chest and breathe slowly through the nose. Hold the position as long as it is comfortable; then go back to the original position lying flat. Repeat three times. You may not complete this posture in the beginning, but go as far as you can. Do not worry even, if you cannot go beyond half-way. The posture must be progressed very slowly to avoid undue strain on the back. After a few months of practice, you will be surprised by your progress.

The plough position can be varied (Plough-variation 1) for more effectiveness by stretching the legs apart as far as possible, keeping the hands firmly on the floor. This stretches the muscles of the legs.

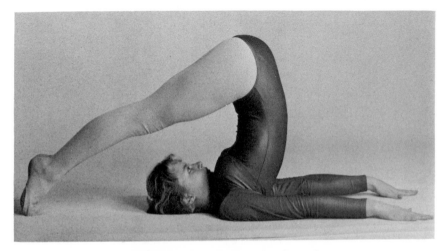

Fig. 8.4. Plough Pose (*Halasana*)

Another variation (Plough-variation 2) gives additional stretching to the lumbar and cervical regions of the spine. Lie down flat with the arms over the head and palms up. Now slowly bring up the legs as in the original plough pose, and touch the hands with the toes.

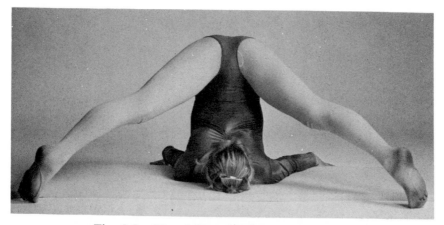

Fig. 8.5.   Plough Pose (*Halasana*)-Variation 1

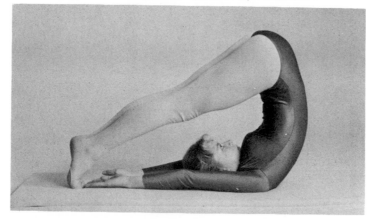

Fig. 8.6.   Plough Pose (*Halasana*)-Variation 2

Ear-knee Pose (Karna Peedasana):   Master the plough position before trying this position. Bring knees down on each side of your head. Put arms around backs of knees and hand over ears. Hold. Return to the plough position and then slowly to the floor.

Forward Bend (Sitting) or Head-knee Pose (Paschimothan Asana):   Sit with the legs outstretched. Raise arms high over head, stretching spine upward and inhaling deeply almost as though yawning. Exhale and bend forward catching toes, if possible. Try to ease the head to the knees. Hold for five seconds and then slowly sit up while inhaling. Repeat three time. If you cannot touch the toes first time, go as far as you can. Increase a little more each day, without straining yourself.

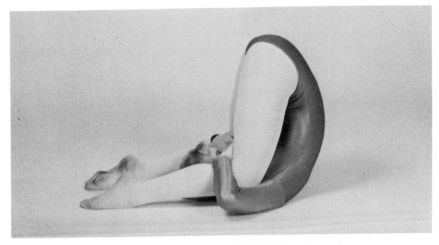

Fig. 8.7.   Ear-knee Pose (*Karna Peedasana*)

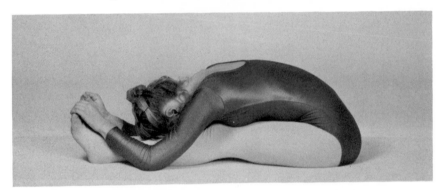

Fig. 8.8.   Head-knee Pose (*Paschimothan Asana*)

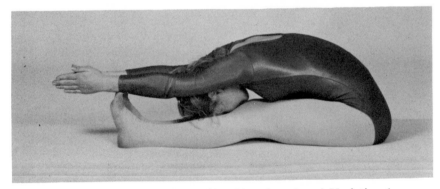

Fig. 8.9.   Head-knee Pose (*Paschimothan Asana*)-Variation 1

Advanced students can practice the above exercise (Head-knee Pose-variation 1) with forehead and nose on the knees and arms extended over the toes or palms flat on the floor.

Another modification of a Head-knee Pose (*Janu Sirasana* Variation 2) is to sit erect with one leg outstretched, the other bent in towards the body so that the heel fits into the crotch, and the sole of the foot presses against the thigh. Gently press the knee to the floor and bend forward, catching the toes of the extended foot. Advanced students should be able to touch the forehead to the knee and press elbows to floor without bending the outstretched leg. Hold five seconds and repeat three times. Repeat on the other side.

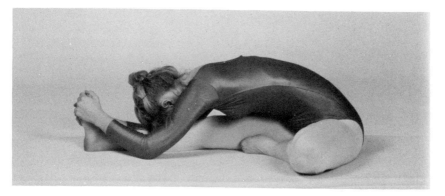

Fig. 8.10.   Head-knee Pose (*Janu Sirasana*)-Variation 2

Backward Bending Exercises: These exercises relieve back pain, tone the abdominal muscles and internal organs, tone the breasts, ovaries and uterus in women, strengthen the neck, and firm jaw line.

Cobra Pose (Bhujangasana):   This exercise is called the cobra pose (*bhujang* means cobra) because the position is in imitation of a cobra about to strike. Lie on your stomach with palms pressing against the floor, fingers forward, fingertips and shoulders in line and legs straight. Successively raise your head, neck, and upper back, keeping the lower half of your body on the floor. Try to feel the motion of the spine rolling back vertebra by vertebra. Retain the pose for a while and slowly bring down your head little by little. Breathe in while you bend backward, hold the breath while in this position, and exhale while coming down. Repeat three to six times. Be careful—not to strain the back muscles by a jerking and wrenching action.

There are many variations of the cobra pose in order to give maximum bending to the spine. In one of the variations (Cobra-variation 1) from the first position, arch the back and straighten the elbows using fingertip pressure.

In a further variation (Cobra-variation 2), bend the spine as much as possible.

Now fold the legs at the knees, bring the toes towards the head, and try to touch the back of the head.

Retaining of pose, breathing sequence, coming down and repeating the exercise are the same in these variations as described for the first position of the cobra pose.

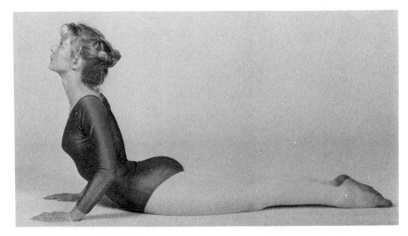

Fig. 8.11. Cobra Pose (*Bhujangasana*)

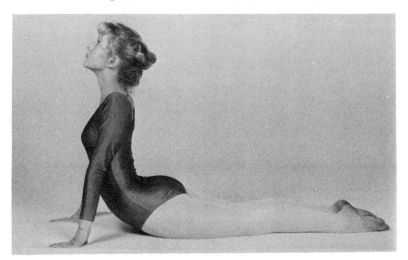

Fig. 8.12. Cobra Pose (*Bhujangasana*)-Variation 1

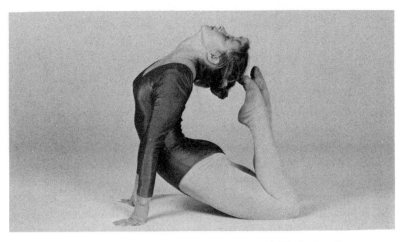

Fig. 8.13. Cobra Pose (*Bhujangasana*)-Variation 2

Locust Pose (Salabhasana):   Lie face down with hands along the sides, palms up. Rest the chin on the ground by raising the head a little. Inhale and raise the left foot, keeping the knee straight and the other leg down. Stretch the leg out and up as far as possible, hold briefly, exhale and lower the leg. Change to the other side and alternate three times on each side. This is the half locust exercise.

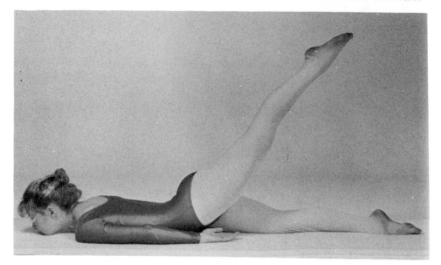

Fig. 8.14.   Locust Pose (*Salabhasana*)

As you progress in the half locust, you can start (Locust-variation 1) lifting both legs simultaneously. Stiffen the whole body and raise the legs high. The knees should be kept straight. Now the chest and the hands will feel the burden of the legs. Keep the thighs, legs, and toes in a straight line. Remain in the pose for fifteen seconds and slowly come down. Repeat three times.

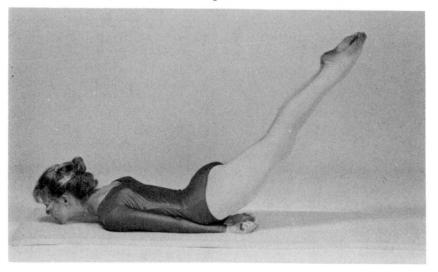

Fig. 8.15.   Locust Pose (*Salabhasana*)-Variation 1

150

After practicing the above position, modify it (Locust-variation 2) by putting more force on the hands to raise the body till the whole body rests on the chin. This exercise, when performed correctly, looks exactly opposite to the shoulder stand (described later).

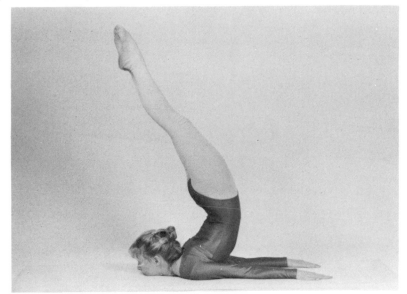

Fig. 8.16.   Locust Pose (*Salabhasana*)-Variation 2

Bow Pose (Dhanurasana):   Lie on your stomach, bend the knees, reach back and catch firm hold of ankles. Inhale and raise your head and knees as though your body was indeed a bow trying to straighten. The pressure of armpull raises the knees from the floor. Advanced students can rock back and forth on the stomach. Repeat three times holding about ten seconds.

Afterward, lie down and catch the left toe with the hand and slowly pull it towards the head, bending the left side of the back (Bow-variation 1). Alternate the procedure for the right side. This can be done two times for each side.

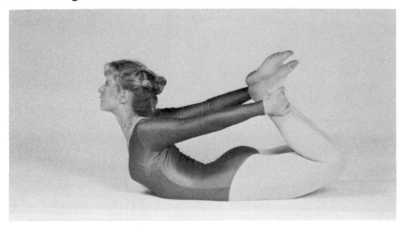

Fig. 8.17.   Bow Pose (*Dhanurasana*)

After the practice of folding one leg at a time in the above pose, lie down on the abdomen and fold both legs at the knees (Bow-variation 2). Take hold of the big toes with the hands and slowly pull the feet toward the head. This gives maximum exercise to the spine.

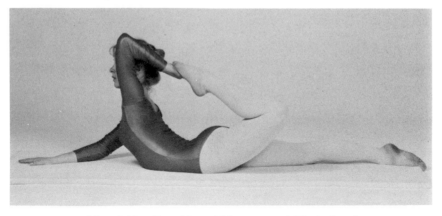

Fig. 8.18. Bow Pose (*Dhanurasana*)-Variation 1

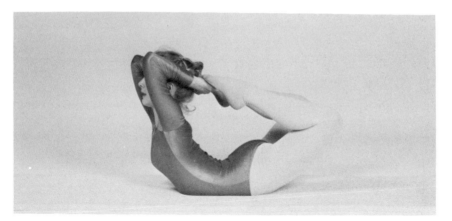

Fig. 8.19. Bow Pose (*Dhanurasana*)-Variation 2

Kneeling Pose (Supta Vajrasana): Sit on the heels with the spine erect. Sliding down, relax shoulders onto the floor and put arms above your head. Hold and try to place your back on the floor. This posture eventually becomes comfortable enough, but be careful at first not to strain the knees.

As a modification of the above pose, rest on the legs and head (Kneeling-variation 1). Keep the hands on the thighs.

For the Full Kneeling Position (*Poorna Supta Vajrasana*-variation 2) sit on the heels and slowly lie down on your back, keeping the knees together. As you touch the floor with your head, lift the buttocks and body from the floor, resting on the head and legs. Use the hands to push your head nearer to the heels.

These postures which stretch the thigh muscles and the abdomen may be used instead of the bow posture for the sake of variety.

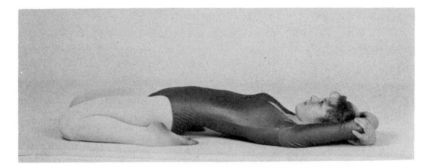

Fig. 8.20.   Kneeling Pose (*Supta Vajrasana*)

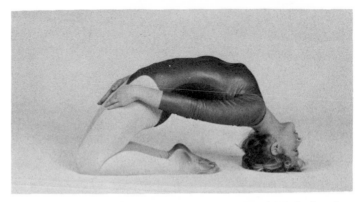

Fig. 8.21.   Kneeling Pose (*Supta Vajrasana*)-Variation 1

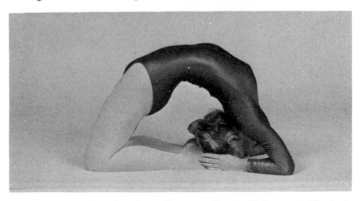

Fig. 8.22.   Full Kneeling Pose (*Poorna Supta Vajrasana*)-Variation 2

Wheel Pose (Chakrasana):   Sit on heels assuming a kneeling position and bend backward, raising the buttocks. Now grasp the ankles. Breathe deeply and hold the breath for a few seconds and repeat three times.

Twisting Exercises: These exercises tone all the spinal nerves, massage the abdominal organs, and are good for constipation and dyspepsia (indigestion).

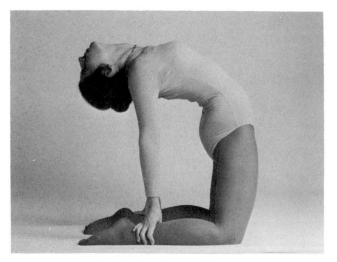

Fig. 8.23. Wheel Pose (*Chakrasana*)

Spinal Twist (Ardha Matsendrasana): Sit with legs outstretched. Bend left leg at the knee and put the right leg underneath the left with the right heel touching the left buttock. Pass the right arm over the left knee and catch hold of the left foot firmly with the right hand and right foot with left hand.

In order to have more mechanical advantage for twisting the spine (Spinal Twist-variation 1), extend the above exercise by swinging the left hand back to catch the right thigh or simply place the left palm behind the hip. Now steadily pull and twist the spine. To help the spine to twist evenly all through, the neck is also turned toward the left shoulder. Repeat, alternating legs and arms.

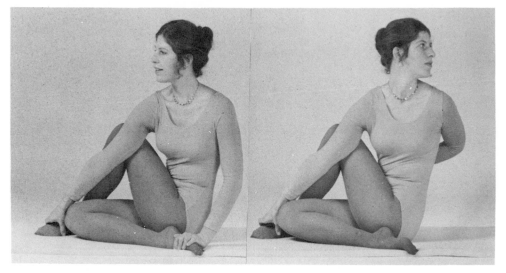

Fig. 8.24. Spinal Twist (*Ardha Matsendrasana*)

Fig. 8.25. Spinal Twist (*Ardha Matsendrasana*)-
Variation 1

To perform another variation of the twisting pose (Spinal Twist-variation 2), sit down. Bend left leg at knee, bringing heel into crotch and keeping knee on ground. Place sole of the right foot on the floor on the left side of the folded left knee. The right knee is bent up to the level of the chest. Now bring the left arm alongside the outer side of the upper raised knee and grasp the left knee. Finally, bring the right arm around the back and grasp the right ankle. At the same time turn your head and look as far around as possible over the right shoulder so that the twist is felt the whole way up the spine and neck. Hold the position half a minute and then reverse the pose.

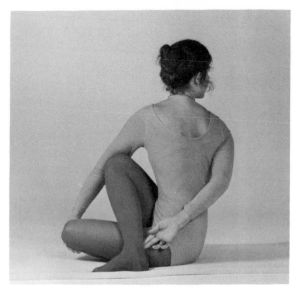

Fig. 8.26.   Spinal Twist (*Ardha Matsendrasana*)-Variation 2

Balancing Exercises: These exercises can help to improve circulation to the brain, relieve sinus congestion, and help with thyroid problems. The aches of head, shoulder, and arms in sedentary workers due to stress on the spine can be relieved by postures, the fish pose and the shoulder stand, which stretch the ligaments and permit free and easy movements of the head and neck.

Shoulder Stand (Sarvangasana):   Lie flat on your back, feet together, and palms on the floor. Inhale, and raise the legs and hips slowly until the whole body attains a vertical position with elbows resting on the floor and both hands supporting the back. Press the chin against the chest. Breathe easily and naturally. Hold the position motionlessly and do not allow the body to shake. Increase gradually to three minutes. When the posture is over, lower the legs very slowly and smoothly. In a further modification (Shoulder Stand-variation 1), the hands that support the body are removed and kept vertically along the body on the thighs. By removing the hands, the whole weight falls on the cervical region and shoulder muscles.

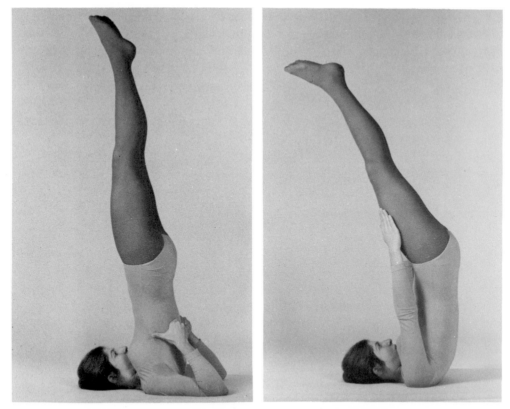

Fig. 8.27. Shoulder Stand (*Sarvangasana*) Fig. 8.28. Shoulder Stand (*Sarvangasana*)-
Variation 1

Bridge Pose (Sethu Bandhasana): Although the Bridge Pose is a separate exercise,
it is often practiced as though it was a variation of the shoulder stand in order to
bend the upper back in an opposite direction and thus reverse the stretching effect.
From the shoulder stand bring down your legs and slowly touch your feet on the
floor. The arms continue to support midback with thumb and fingers spread
about the waist. Practice switching from the shoulder stand to the bridge and
back again.

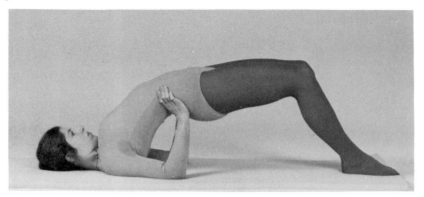

Fig. 8.29. Bridge Pose (*Sethu Bandhasana*)

Fish Pose (Matsyasana): For beginners, lie on your back. Stretch legs and keep the hands down under the buttocks with palms facing the floor or vice versa. Raise the chest with the help of the elbows and bend the neck backward as much as possible. Rest on the top of the head.

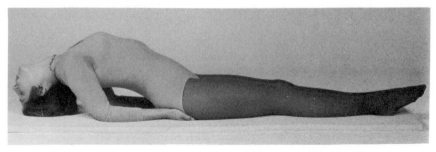

Fig. 8.30.   Fish Pose (*Matsyasana*)

For the classic fish pose (Fish-variation 1), sit in a lotus posture (if the lotus appears difficult use the easy pose by simply crossing the legs). Lie on the back. Rest the elbows on the floor. Now lift the trunk and rest the top of the head on the floor by bending the back and neck. Then catch hold of the toes.

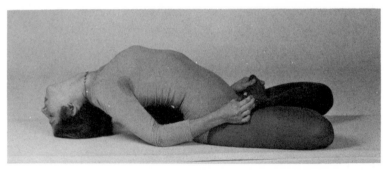

Fig. 8.31.   Fish Pose (*Matsyasana*)-Variation 1

In another position of the fish (Fish-variation 2), the chest is thrown open with the arms crossed behind your head. Hold the position as long as it is comfortable and breathe deeply. The fish can follow the shoulder stand to give an opposite stretch.

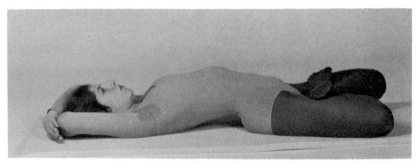

Fig. 8.32.   Fish Pose (*Matsyasana*)-Variation 2

Headstand (Sirshasana): Kneel down and clasp hands with the fingers lightly interlocked and the back of the head resting between the hands. The top of the head touches the floor, but all the weight is distributed along the arms and elbows, which press solidly down. The top of the head may be supported from behind by the fingerlock. With the help of toes and knees when the trunk is sufficiently thrown back, you can slowly remove the toes from the floor. Slowly raise the legs high up in the air till the whole body becomes erect. By regularly practicing you can increase the time for holding the pose from five seconds up to fifteen minutes. Instead of a fingerlock method, you can keep the palms of your hands on the blanket on each side. However, you may find it easier to do against the wall or some other suitable support. After completing the posture lower the legs slowly to the original position and stand erect for a minute or two. This will harmonize the blood circulation.

The headstand and other upside-down postures like the shoulder stand are very important for a rich supply of blood to the brain. Daily practice of these exercises for 10 to 15 minutes increases the memory and intellectual power, as well as the supply of blood to the upper parts of the back, the neck, eyes, and ears. Upside-down postures also help the return of blood to the heart from regions below its level. The head stand is a good exercise for strengthening the vertebral column. Hanging upside-down on a bar using an ankle-lock (a new American health practice) is based on similar principles. It helps to increase blood supply to the brain, and to straighten and relax the spinal column for those with back problems. Persons with health conditions like high blood pressure should not attempt upside-down exercises.

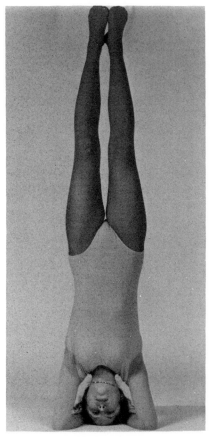

Fig. 8.33. Headstand (*Sirshasana*)

Yogic Exercises for Leg Joints and Feet: These exercises help to strengthen ankle and knee joints and tighten thigh muscles. Walking bare-footed, whenever possible is also a good exercise for feet.

Frog Pose (Mandukasana): Sit in a kneeling position keeping the feet and knees together, and the spine erect. Now separate the knees as far apart as possible. Sit firmly on the floor and place the hands on the knees. Sit in this pose for one to three minutes.

Cow Head Pose (Gomukhasana): In this position, the ankle twist is opposite of the frog position. The heels are kept sideways with the toes pointing away from the body, giving an extra twist to the knee joints. Sitting comfortably raise your left hand and bring it behind your shoulder. Now bend the right hand behind the back from the bottom and stretch diagonally upward until fingers interlock. Repeat, with right arm reaching back over right shoulder. You can do the arm phase of the exercise by standing up; this will keep shoulders supple and help prevent bursitis.

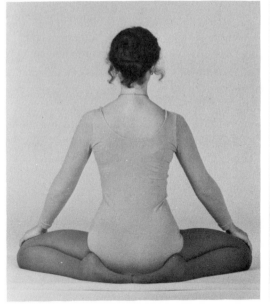 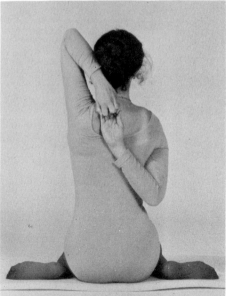

Fig. 8.34. Frog Pose (*Mandukasana*)   Fig. 8.35. Cow Head Pose (*Gomukhasana*)

Dog Pose: Lie down on your stomach with palms pressing against the floor as in the cobra pose. Exhale and lift the body. Keep the feet and heels flat on the floor. Now walk forward as much as you can trying to keep the legs straight. Now raise and lower your heels together without moving your palms. Repeat five times.

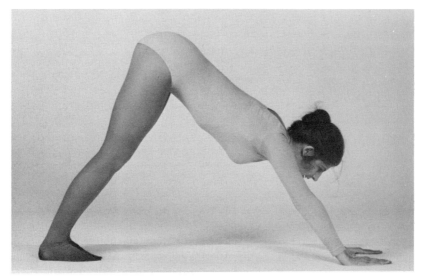

Fig. 8.36.   Dog Pose

Meditative Positions (Sitting Postures):   These postures are good for breathing exercises and meditation purposes. Use any of the positions given below whichever is the most comfortable for you so long as you keep the body erect. An uncomfortable position will take your concentration away from breathing and meditation.

Easy Pose (Sukhasana):   The easy pose is a simple, comfortable position. Legs are either folded comfortably that suits an individual or crossed in front with knees resting on insteps. Head, neck and trunk should be in a line without any curve.

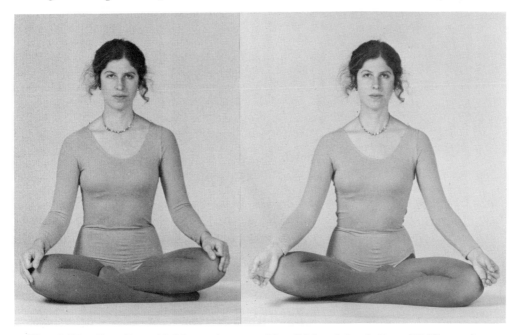

Fig. 8.37.   Easy Pose (*Sukhasana*)   Fig. 8.38.   Adept's Pose (*Siddhasana*)

Adept's or Perfect Pose (Siddhasana):   In the sitting position, the legs are bent inward to the crotch with soles turned upward. The heel of one foot rests on top of the heel of the other in such a way that both heels fit comfortably into the crotch. The knees should touch the floor and the back should remain erect with hands resting on the knees. The position is used by the great saints and yogis for longterm sitting.

Lotus Pose (Padamasana):   Take hold of your right foot, folding the leg at the knee to place the foot on the left thigh. Similarly, fold the left leg and place it on the right thigh. Soles should turn upward with knees remaining on the floor. Keep your back straight and place your hands over your knees with thumb and fore-finger making a circle and last three fingers extended.

Ankle Lock (Swastikasana):   This position is worth mastering for the beginners who find the lotus a difficult position. In this modified lotus, the feet are not pulled back as high as in the lotus but snuggle against the inner thigh.

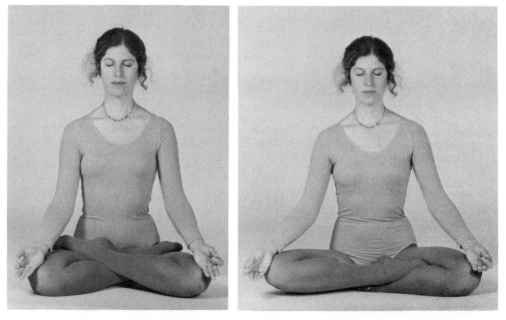

Fig. 8.39.   Lotus Pose (*Padamasana*)   Fig. 8.40.   Ankle Lock (*Swastikasana*)

Yoga Exercises for Throat, Tongue and Gas in the Stomach: The Lion Pose can help to increase circulation to the tongue and throat. The wind relieving pose can help people with indigestion and other abdominal ailments.

Lion Pose (Simhasana):   Assume a kneeling position, keeping palms on the knees. Lean over the hands. Now protrude the tongue as far as possible by contracting the throat muscles. Try to role your eyeballs upward. The whole body is stiffened as though the lion is about to jump upon its prey. During this position exhale the breath as much as possible. Repeat four to six times.

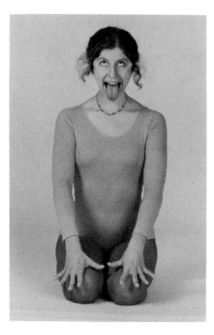

Fig. 8.41.   Lion Pose (*Simhasana*)

Wind Relieving Pose (Vatayanasana):   Lie flat on your back. Now inhale deeply and hold your breath. While you are holding your breath, fold your left leg at the knee and press the folded leg against the abdomen. Use both hands to get the maximum pressure. Keep the right leg straight. Repeat three times with each leg alternately. Now use both legs and press both knees against the abdomen, three times, as for one leg.

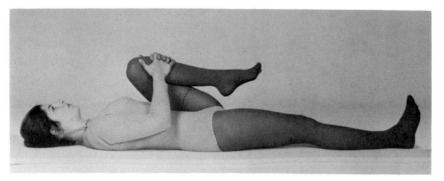

Fig. 8.42.   Wind Relieving Pose (*Vatayanasana*)

Relaxation Posture (*Savasana*):   This posture restores energy and relieves tension.
    Lie flat on your back with the feet slightly apart, arms along sides, and palms up. Quiet yourself and keep the body loose. Close your eyes and relax muscle by muscle from the head downward to the toes, breathing in slowly and deeply from the diaphragm. Then follow the same course but now tensing each muscle group. Finally, have a good overall stretch.

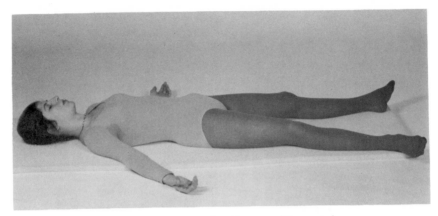

Fig. 8.43.   Relaxation Posture (*Savasana*)

Eye Exercises: These help to relieve eye strain, strengthen eye muscles, and may even improve eyesight. These can also help to develop concentration and mental focusing.

Gazing (Tratak):   Keep a candle flame or similar object three to four feet away from your body. The level of your eyes and the candle flame should be in a horizontal line. Sit erect in one of the meditative positions, keeping the spine straight and the body relaxed. For one minute look upon the flame with a steady gaze and without winking. Alternately, you can look in your own eyes in the mirror for a minute without winking. After a minute close the eyes and relax the eye muscles. Gradually increase the period of gazing from one to three minutes, spending equal time relaxing the eyes.

Nasal Gaze (Nasagra):   Sit in a comfortable position with you body relaxed and gaze at the tip of your nose for one or two minutes. Repeat practice and relaxation (by closing your eyes) several times.

Eye Twisting Exercises: Work on the eye exercises given below gradually. Sitting in a comfortable position, look as far as possible to the right moving only the eyes. Then to the left. Alternate five times and close ten seconds to rest. Repeat similarly by raising and lowering eyes, with a diagonal motion-up right and down left. Reverse. Close the eyes and rest.

   During the above exercises, resting of the eyes can be accomplished by resting the palms of your hands on closed eyelids with the fingers pointing up.

Nasal Cleaning (*Neti*):   In addition to normal daily hygiene the nasal passages should be washed out with lukewarm salt water. The regular cleaning of the nasal passages is an excellent preventive measure for colds and sore throats because the mucous membranes are strengthened. Breathing becomes easier; therefore it is preferable to do breathing exercises after this cleaning. It also helps to strengthen the eyes because the blood vessels of the eye are stimulated.

To one pint of lukewarm water add a teaspoonful of common salt; this has the salt content close to that of tears. One method is that the salted water is cupped in the hand and sniffed up each nostril and then expelled by blowing out, first of one nostril and then of the other. Doing this two to three times should be sufficient to clear the nasal passages.

There is another method using nasal douche which may be obtained at a drug store. With the use of a nasal douche, pour a small portion of the salted water through one nostril, closing the other with the thumb. Raise the head and allow the water to flow down to the mouth, then spit it out. Repeat this process two or more times with each nostril. At this point, a small quantity of water will remain in the nasal passage, which must be blown out by a forced expiration; this can be accomplished by blocking one nostril and exhaling vigorously through the other. If you feel pressure on your ears while blowing out the water, keep your mouth open.

Stomach Cleaning (*Dhauti*)?: In addition to nose, another major area that requires special attention is the stomach. According to yoga system, these two areas are of special significance, for they are the vehicles for the important functions of breathing and eating, fundamental to sustaining life. One of the simple stomach cleaning techniques (*dhauti*), commonly described in yoga books, is water purification. Drink a large quantity of salt water and shake the abdominal portions. Contract the stomach and put the fingers at the root of the tongue and tickle until the water is vomited or thrown out. Rather than trying this unusual technique, I would suggest the prevention technique of using the right kind of food and occasional fast to keep the stomach clean and healthy. Stomach care or cleaning becomes necessary only when we eat large quantities of wrong foods, such as high fat, excessive protein, and lots of salt, pepper, mustard, vinegar, pickles, or other condiments. By avoiding these foods, one would not only have a clean stomach but also clean kidneys.

Note: In this chapter, we have touched the important aspects of yoga which are to keep the whole person clean and fit. After performing the postures and exercises many people feel relaxed physically as well as mentally. Posture is that which is steady, stable, and firm as well as easy and pleasant. There are many more complex postures than the ones in this chapter. But it is unwise to waste time on contortions, especially when simpler exercises confer similar benefits. We should also remember that yoga is not a set of practices, but a way of life that is part of the everyday world, We must learn the art of touching the world lightly; moderation in everything, extremism in nothing. If one maintains the proper attitudes, there is no need to speak or act excessively or elaborately. When one learns this beautiful practice, his presence will touch everyone around him, for he will leave an indelible mark on others souls. This is the only print that a true believer of yoga leaves when he departs.

Chapter 9

Concluding Remarks

Nature is logical in all ways. No exceptions. Albert Einstein phrases the same thing in a different way, "I shall never believe that God plays dice with the world." Do things nature's way and you have something powerful going for you. Depart from nature, and terrible things must be printed after the word "caution" on medicine bottles. Even the most orthodox medical scientist will eventually have to come to terms with a simple, safe therapy which makes so many of the tired energetic, the old younger, and the sick well.

We have been progressing in technologies, sciences, hypotheses, discoveries, but we are hopelessly ignorant about problems of everyday life, including health. In spite of our achievements in education, material wealth, organized society and security through insurances of all kinds, cases of fear and anxiety, worry and depression, insecurity, violence, and sickness are still rising. Health professionals are in higher demand than ever, and hospital facilities are still expanding. As we all know, medicine is a disease care program rather than a health care program. We are in such desperate need of a disease care program only because we ignore a health care program. One is born to be healthy and not to be sick. Good health is a natural state of the human body. In this book we have discussed maintaining this state—and restoring it if it is lost—in ways that are natural to the body—not with powerful drugs, but with natural healthy activities including wholesome natural foods.

Our state of well-being or feeling good depends on the amount of energy available to us. More energy available to our brain cells should make us feel brighter. More energy available to all our cells should make us feel not only energetic, but also resistant to many diseases. For example, we know that people who are malnourished have a tremendously decreased resistance to diseases. In the last several years there has been an exciting development of interest in ways to help us avoid sickness, feel more energetic, and to live life to the fullest. Notable among these ways are the bioenergetics movement, transcendental meditation, group therapy, nutrition, breathing exercises, yoga and other exercise programs.

As you must have realized by now, the main intention in this book has been to utilize these programs for increasing the body's natural ability to produce more energy by following natural safe daily activities along with breathing exercises, yoga, and wholesome natural foods. These practical steps are not gimmicks but something that can be incorporated into a daily life style and stay with us for the rest of our lives. The degree of change to be felt will depend upon one's present health, and the degree of adherence to these habits. As a reminder about some of the important steps, a summary of recommended activities is reemphasized in the following pages.

Life Attitudes

Everyone wants health and happiness. However, few of us put forth efforts to change our daily life attitudes and take care of ourselves. The following points suggest behavior modifications aimed at restoring positive mental attitudes. (The Desiderata quotes, wherever used, are given in quotation marks.)

1. Happiness is a matter of setting personal standards, and not chasing after other people's. "If you compare yourself with others, you may become vain and bitter; for always there will be greater and lesser persons than yourself. Keep interested in your own career, however humble; it is a real possession in the changing fortunes of time."

2. Maintain a balance between expectations and achievements. Unrealistic expectations can lead towards frustration. Have a goal which you can hope to attain. If it is too high it will result in discouragement if you fail. When you succeed you can then raise the standard, step by step. "Enjoy your achievements as well as your plans."

3. Work is good for you. Do not avoid work but find the kind that suits you the best. Hard workers in almost any field often live to a very advanced age.

4. Comfort weakens us, and difficulty strengthens us. When we seek comfort, comfort produces ease, ease produces weakness, weakness produces poverty, and poverty produces difficulty. So a seeking of comfort ends by producing difficulty. To end difficulty, we seek comfort again. Thus, comfort is not a key to end difficulties and to bring happiness. Whenever there is no difficulty, there is no development.

5. The people we call enemies can be good for us. The enemy who accuses and attacks us, makes us cautious in action, deliberate in thought and stronger in our abilities. On the other hand, if we live with only the friends who give us sweet words of consolation and loving supportive care we become weaker.

6. The people who irritate us because of their sarcastic, deceptive, jealous, or egotistical behavior need help. Our calmness towards their behavior would help them and in return would bring us satisfaction from doing a good deed.

7. It is a relative world with tops and bottoms, riches and poors, strongs and weaks. We can reach the top of the mountain only if we are not there (and sitting somewhere at the foot or middle of the mountain). When we are at the bottom of society—with our ambitious and adventurous spirit—we can eventually attain the top of society, and it is the striving that brings us satisfaction.

8. We should not be afraid of failure and stay behind people to protect us. If we stay at a low level, we never experience falling down. Remember,

you face failure only when you try for achievement. It is not a crime to fail—the sin is to have a low aim.

9. Although accomplishments and active living itself requires some stress, living under constant stressful conditions is dangerously harmful. Try to reduce stress by avoiding stressful environments through physical activity or more progressively through mental approaches as emphasized in Chapter 2.

10. Constructive assessment of your mistakes and short-comings is a healthy step, but calling yourself names, or expressing frustration at your limitations create a negative emotional effect on your body.

11. Remember that worry, anxiety and fear will not solve any problem. If there is a problem, collect the facts, then ask yourself what is the worst possible result that can happen, and decide to accept even this if necessary. Dismiss the problem from your mind but keep the hope and the expectation of a good result.

12. Although a certain amount of earnings is a necessity and money does provide some freedom, true happiness exists in the head, not the wallet. Therefore, those who use money as a vehicle towards happiness are highly unlikely to be successful. The race for money usually leaves people hollow and dissatisfied.

13. Self-motivation may lead one to realize that life has some meaning and direction. An active life—having a reason for living is a healthy attitude.

14. "Realize that sham, drudgery and broken dreams are a part of life, it is still a beautiful world. Strive to be happy."

15. Efforts should be made to kick out feelings of inhibition to make place for enthusiasm. Life is a balance between enthusiasm and inhibition. If enthusiasm dominates inhibition, life can be full of liveliness and satisfaction, but if inhibition dominates, life will be empty.

16. Be temperate in all things. Avoid extremes. Take a more detached view of life, neither over-elated by success nor depressed by failure.

17. Have a plan for each day, but do not be a slave to the plan.

18. Think before you act. A wrong thought can be rectified more quickly than a wrong action. When questioned, think and then reply; try not to jump to conclusions.

19. Have a positive attitude to everything you do or think about. Negative attitudes invite failure.

20. Think about other people rather than about yourself. Do not be a cause of injury to others. Be compassionate. Forgive the weaknesses of others.

21. "As far as possible, without surrender, be on good terms with all persons. Speak your truth quietly and clearly; and listen to others, even the dull and ignorant. They too have their story."

22. Learn to withdraw into an inner privacy of mind even in the thickest crowd.

23. "Avoid loud and aggressive persons, they are vexatious to the spirit."

24. "Be yourself. Especially do not feign affection. Neither be cynical about love; for in the face of all aridity and disenchantment it is perennial as the grass."

25. "You are a child of the universe, no less than the trees and the stars; you have a right to be here. Therefore be at peace with God, whatever you conceive him to be, and whatever the labors and aspirations, in the noisy confusion of life keep peace with your soul."

Nutrition and Eating Habits

Sixtyfive percent of deaths over the age of sixtyfive occur due to heart-related problems, 21% due to cancer and 14% due to other causes. The overall death rate for all age groups from heart ailments, stroke, and cancer account for 75% of deaths in the United States. Fortunately, this higher death rate, which is primarily due to our own careless habits, can be reduced. Nutrition is one of the most effective means to reduce the risks of serious health problems. For example, careful nutrition can reduce the risk of heart-related diseases either directly by lowering cholesterol intake or indirectly by controlling weight through proper eating habits. Some of the important dietary principles are listed below.

1. Eat three regular meals a day and include breakfast regularly. However, do not eat just because it is a meal-time unless you feel you need food. Eat a variety of foods, so that you get proteins, carbohydrates, fats, minerals and vitamins.

2. Fat children with a high number of fat cells usually grow as fat adults. Therefore, it is very important to introduce youngsters to nutritionally sound eating habits. Normally an average weight person rarely becomes obese in later life (after, say, the age of 30).

3. Maintain an ideal weight. People with normal or slightly below normal weight live longer than those who are overweight.

4. If you consume more calories than you use—whether from protein, carbohydrate, or fat—you will gain weight. The extra calories are always converted to fat and accumulate in the body as fat, no matter what their source is—a carrot or a steak or a piece of bread or a spoonful of butter. Consumption of 3,500 extra Calories means a pound of body fat.

5. Repeated gaining, losing, and regaining of extra pounds is more damaging to your health than just remaining overweight. That is why it is important to give up the notion of a "diet." A diet is something you go on and off. Permanent weight control means an eating plan that is the same today and a year from today and for the rest of your life.

6. "Don't diet" is becoming the newest slogan, and a step in the right direction. Every fad diet, we know so far, is nutritionally unbalanced in one way or another, and some are downright dangerous, even if followed by healthy people for a relatively short time. The weight-loss products such as diet pills generally cause temporary water loss and do not provide a weight-loss solution. Moreover, the side effects can be very serious. The only permanent solution for weight reduction is to maintain a caloric balance by cutting food calories sensibly or by burning calories through physical activity.

7. To maintain proper weight and good health, consume plenty of foods such as whole-wheat bread and rolls, oatmeal, brown rice, sprouts, legumes (beans, peas, lentils), fresh fruits and vegetables, milk and milk products (low-fat). But avoid fats, oils, sugars and syrups, fat milk, fried foods, egg yolk, alcoholic beverages, and canned fruits with added sugars.

8. Unfortunately, most overweight people like the fattening foods which made them overweight in the first place. To change your habit of liking healthy foods instead of fattening foods, eat healthy foods when hungry and the fattening foods only when you are less hungry. This will help you in developing gradually a taste for healthy over junk foods. Although it is difficult to immediately change eating habits, with persistence you can gradually increase the amount of healthy foods over undesirable fattening and unhealthy foods.

9. Once you learn to live normally with food, you don't have to exercise for the sake of maintaining a normal weight. Low calorie wholesome foods will naturally help maintain caloric balance. Lack of exercise is not itself a cause of overweight.

10. In general, the less fat you eat of any type, the better. But whenever possible, use vegetable oils in place of hard shortenings and animal fats.

11. Limit protein intake from animal sources. Remember, only foods from animal sources are rich in cholesterol, a prime factor in coronary artery disease. In case you include animal protein, the species that are more primordial should be preferred over highly evolved ones. This means fowl such as chicken or turkey is recommended over mammals such as beef and pork; fish and other seafood are even more suitable than fowl. Excess protein is of no use to the body except as an energy source, in other words, calories. So you can get fat eating too much protein.

12. Carbohydrates are no more fattening than protein, and should be consumed in sufficient quantity for providing energy.

13. It is hard to be a fat vegetarian. To reduce weight, increase the amount of vegetarian foods. With proper combinations vegetarian foods can provide most of the necessary amino acids. In fact, vegetarian foods such as grains, roots, vegetables, and fruits in an unrefined, minimally processed form are among the best sources for protein.

14. Vegetarian foods provide adequate amounts of fiber, minerals, and vitamins, and are almost lacking in fat and cholesterol.

15. Avoid adding commercially sold fiber to your food. Good sources of fiber are fruits, vegetables, and whole grains. Sufficient addition of these foods to daily diet should alleviate constipation and intestinal disorders.

16. Vegetarians eating no animal protein at all may require supplement of vitamin B_{12} once every several weeks. However, vegetarians who include milk and milk products in their diet get B_{12} supply from milk and its products.

17. Synthetic and natural vitamins are chemically the same and perform the same function. However, vitamins from natural foods are less concentrated

and are accompanied by other nutrients which share metabolic reactions to give the full nutritional effect.

18. Over-cooking can destroy heat sensitive vitamins such as vitamin C, B_1 and pantothenic acid.

19. Too much consumption of fat soluble vitamins A, D, E, and K, may result in excessive accumulation of these vitamins in the body, and thus may cause serious side effects. Excessive amounts of water soluble vitamins, B-complex and C, however, are excreted from the body.

20. Milk is an excellent source of high quality protein, calcium and several other useful nutrients for children and adults. However, in people with low production of the enzyme lactase, the milk sugar (lactose) cannot be broken down into glucose and galactose and causes a problem, sometimes an allergic reaction to undigested milk protein. So milk is a perfect food for most people, but unfortunately not for everyone.

21. The use of sugar, salt, alcohol, and caffeine should be reduced to a minimum. Smoking is undoubtedly dangerous to health, and should obviously be avoided.

22. Try to understand the nutritional values of food and—without becoming a diet freak—keep in mind the effects of various foods on your health.

23. Simultaneous availability of all the necessary amino acids (units of a protein) is needed for the synthesis of a particular protein that may be required for the structure of body tissues, proper body functioning, or disease resistance. Knowledge about the combination of foods is, therefore, important to ensure the supply of all the necessary amino acids, as emphasized in Chapter 5. It is important to remember that people do not have to depend on meat for protein and the correct supply of amino acids. By using the proper combination, the necessary amino acids can be obtained from a vegetarian diet, thus avoiding the risks associated with higher meat consumption.

24. Do not eat immediately before or after exercise or immediately after physical work or a hurried walk.

25. Do not involve yourself in hard mental work for at least 15 minutes before and after meals. If tired, relax for 10–15 minutes before eating. Pleasant conversation or relaxed thinking while eating is good; arguing or concentrating on the day's problems is harmful.

26. Drinking pure water with food helps digestion. However, cut down drinking of water at meal times; drink about half an hour before or after a meal. Fruit juices are best, but fresh made tea will cause no harm.

27. It is important to avoid overeating. Try to stop eating when the appetite is about 80% satisfied. Occasional fasting is useful; if possible, once a month is suggested.

28. Cleaning the mouth before and after meals is a healthful habit and keeps teeth healthy.

29. Slow eating is a good habit and helps in digestion. Food should be taken into the system no faster than it can be thoroughly communicated by the

teeth. Proper mastication by teeth saves the stomach from an extra burden.

30. Mastication and slow eating help to maintain a proper weight by diminishing any sensation of abnormal appetite.

31. Fruit, whole grains, and raw vegetables—essentials of a good vegetarian diet—take a lot more chewing than meat and white bread. Besides being helpful to stimulate secretion of saliva and gastric juices, which aid digestion, chewing is important for healthy teeth.

32. The caloric intake for individuals over 50 years of age should be reduced to 90 percent of the amount required by a mature adult. In other words, a person consuming 3,000 Calories would need to reduce his intake to about 2,700 Calories.

Preventive Measures and Physical Fitness

Medical advances have tamed the killer diseases of the past such as polio, tuberculosis and other infectious diseases. However, in increasing numbers, people are killing themselves from preventable cause such as smoking, poor diet, heart problems and cancer. The following points emphasize some measures which help to maintain physical fitness and prevent degenerative health problems.

1. Excessive use of certain foods such as sugar, salt, red meat, fat and cholesterol can be a leading factor in many of the deadly ailments. Most heart troubles result from animal food and other food containing saturated fat, sugar and other sweeteners causing formation of fatty acids, or excessive liquid including alcoholic beverages. Moderation in eating these foods, therefore, is simply logical.

2. To avoid constipation and other intestinal ailments eat foods with adequate amounts of roughage. As a healthy step, increase the use of whole grains, cereals, fruits, vegetables and legumes.

3. To reduce the risks of cancer consume fruits and vegetables rich in vitamin C (e.g. citrus fruits, tomatoes, and peppers) and beta-carotene, a precursor of vitamin A (e.g. dark green leaf vegetables such as spinach and broccoli and deep-yellow fruits and vegetables such as carrots). Also consume the vegetables in the cabbage family, such as cauliflower, kale, brussels and broccoli, which contain natural cancer-inhibiting substances. Fruits and vegetables along with whole grains also help to reduce risks of cancer by providing high proportion of dietary fiber. Avoid high-fat diets, such as fatty meats and other fat and oil sources. High fat consumption is linked to cancers of the colon, breast and prostate. (National Research Council recommends that proportion of calories in the diet provided by fat be reduced from 40 percent to 30 percent.)

4. The consumption of salt-cured, salt-pickled, and smoked foods such as sausages, smoked fish and ham, bacon, and hot dogs should be minimized, because these are associated with increased incidence of stomach and esophagus cancers. Excessive consumption of alcohol, particularly in combination with cigarette smoking should be avoided, because, such consump-

tion has been associated with an increased risk of cancer of the upper gastrointestinal and respiratory tracts.

5. Food is creating us. In a very literal biochemical sense, "we are what we eat." When we choose our daily food and drink, we should keep in mind whether they are really proper to produce the best quality of blood and cells to secure our best mental and physical conditions. The proper practice of dietary habits will be indicated by such symptoms as reduced sickness, sound mentality, and endurance for hardship.

6. Breathe in the pure fresh air as much as possible, whether in the house or outside, sick or healthy. Modern heating and air-conditioning systems increase the extent to which we breathe old stagnant air. Use these to a minimum. By opening windows in the morning or late evening during summer, for instance, you will not only get fresh air, but will save on energy too.

7. To avoid unpleasant odors, do not produce another odor by using sprays. It is far better to provide a supply of fresh air than to fill your lungs with artificial chemicals.

8. Rich supply of oxygen increases the body's energy production and thus enhances both physical and mental well-being. Therefore, increase your oxygen intake by filling your lungs with air to their full capacity. For this purpose utilize low, mid and high breathing as explained in Chapter 7.

9. Do not contract the abdominal muscles during breathing. Note that the stomach moves out and in during inhalation and exhalation, respectively. The movements of the stomach would indicate utilization of diaphragm (the muscular partition between thoracic and abdominal cavity) that increases breathing capacity as explained in Chapter 7.

10. Regular breathing exercises can help to cure pulmonary, cardiac, dropsical, and asthma diseases. Breathing practices can relieve fatigue and anxiety, and can be used to replace such harmful stimulants as coffee and smoking. A rich supply of oxygen to the brain can correct a tired, cranky or moody state of mind. Breathing can be used to induce restful sleep. Remember that sleeping aids decrease the ability to dream, thus blocking an important natural mechanism for relieving stress on a day to day basis.

11. Breathing capacity, which decreases with age can be maintained by proper breathing exercises as given in Chapter 7. Breathing exercises also help to prevent age-related awakenings in older people due to breathing disturbances.

12. Bodily exercise is required of all, whether high or low, rich or poor, in order to promote health and strength. Any physical activity is good for weight control. However, irregular exercise will be of little benefit to total body fitness. Irregular and strenuous exercises can be dangerous. Exercise at better than 50% of your capacity for about 15 to 30 minutes at least three times a week. If it is too much for you—don't worry—select the alternative approaches of walking and yoga as discussed below.

13. It is better to exercise moderately in the morning before eating and if

possible in the open air. Violent exercise should never be performed either immediately before or after eating. Wait for an hour after eating.

14. If you do not enjoy jogging and strenuous exercises, don't push yourself. Walking and yogic exercises are even better and more revitalizing, and may fit more smoothly into your daily life.

15. Walking may not cure everything, you understand, but it is one of the best cures of all. It helps the blood circulation, soothes nervous tension, relieves anxiety, and eases frustration. Walking after dinner helps to ensure a good sleep, especially for sedentary workers.

16. Walking can be maintained with less effort than any other exercises. For example, for a short distance make a habit of walking rather than using a car or bus.

17. Yogic exercises differ from other physical exercises because of the slow movements of joints and muscles involved. The stretching of muscles and ligaments relaxes them and carries more energy to the muscle fibers. Stretched blood vessels help circulation and an equitable flow of blood to various parts of the body.

18. Yogic exercises keep the body flexible, help arthritis, and prevent common back problems.

19. Physical activity and sufficient calcium intake (e.g. by sufficient consumption of milk) can help in maintaining age-related bone mass decrease.

20. Free radicals produced naturally by cells or from exposure to chemicals or nuclear fall outs or X-rays can promote aging. Antioxidants such as vitamins E and C may slow down such free radical damage.

At the end, this whole book might have left you wondering why the approaches discussed are so simple and so inexpensive, compared to advanced and expensive medical approaches. However, you must realize that these approaches are based on centuries of experiences according to the laws of nature, which of course, are evaluated in view of modern scientific knowledge, wherever possible. We know that nature is simple, logical and economical. For example, parts of body not used have been reduced or eliminated through evolutionary processes of nature; our energy machine developed by nature is far more efficient than any gas, diesel, jet or electrical energy machine developed so far. Although we are making great advances in medical research and health technology, we see at the same time more people suffering with sickness, physical and mental, because we have moved away from nature. Many large hospital facilities are fully crowded with patients, more medical insurances are bought than ever before, and many drugstores on every corner are visited from morning till evening by a constant stream of people. It is also important to note that these problems are not confined to a particular place, but to the entire world.

To achieve a fully peaceful world, the constructive development of—not one person, or one city or one state or one nation—but of whole human society is required. We live in a global society within which it is possible for everyone to enjoy health, freedom and happiness. We must begin with the recovery of the physical and mental health of every person, family and community by the establishment of the wholesome health of each individual through the preventive practices of nature's way.

In addition to keeping up with the modern era of advances in science and technology, we should learn how to maintain our health (in view of Eastern as well as Western approaches) and what to do when we become sick. We should have a knowledge of daily health activities which fit naturally into our lives and that include dietary practices, mental attitude, and physical fitness. Health, happiness, and longevity is the endless realization of our infinite dream.

Future Note: Research on the effects of food and nutrients on human behavior is gaining serious attention. There is good biochemical evidence that in laboratory animals, changes in the diet can change the amount of various neurotransmitters synthesized in the brain and can there by alter behavior. The preliminary studies strongly indicate that the same phenomena occur in humans. Scientific experiments have established that several amino derivatives (vitamin B-complex, some amino acids or alcohols) are required for building neurotransmitters, which regulate functioning of the nervous system. Richard Wurtman and his associates of Massachusetts Institute of Technology (MIT) and others have found that half a dozen chemicals such as serotonin, dopamine, norepinephrine, acetylcholine, histamine, and glycine can alter the synthesis of the nerurotransmitters and thus the mental performance of an individual. Shortages of neurotransmitters can cause a loss of memory, depression and senility.

In addition to neurotransmitters, the studies are concentrating on biochemicals that can positively affect such activities as immunity, sleelp problems and sex drive. Scientist are also testing chemicals that can save one from age related damage, can reduce serum cholesterol and can be effective against killer diseases such as cancer. These chemicals, natural as well as synthetic, are further related to particular foods, and it seems plausible that diet may play a very important role in affecting human behavior and health.

The best studied behavioral effect of nutrients in humans is sleepiness. Researchers have suggested that the high carbohydrate meal influence brain tryptophan level and can make mildly insomniac patients fall asleep more quickly and wake less frequently during the night. In view of these results, Michael Yogman of Harvard Medical School strongly suspects that variation in carbohydrate content of breast milk may affect the brain tryptophan level, and therefore, influences the sleep patterns of breast-fed babies. Old remedy of warm milk before bed is a good example of nutrient effect on our behavior.

Although the studies on the effects of nutrients on human behavior have barely begun, there is no longer any real controversy over whether nutrients can affect our behavior. Researcher have begun to ask whether eating breakfast high in protein or high in carbohydrate affect our performance. They have begun to suggest combinations of lecithin, wheat germ, yeast, and linoleate oil (or sunflower seeds) for atherosclerosis, arthritis, and other problems; and carbohydrate rich foods such as cookies and pasta for depression, to name a few.

Appendix A

Natural-Vegetarian Diet Recipes

The following pages include both low calorie and gourmet recipes, mostly of wholesome natural foods. Many of the low calorie recipes (50 to 100 Calories per serving) that are very effective for weight loss are marked'*'. The choice of recipes depends on personal preference and individual weight requirements. You must keep in mind that for fancy gourmet foods you have to pay a price in greater calorie and fat consumption. It will be wise to enjoy fancy foods occasionally rather than every day. The low calorie recipes are very effective for losing or controlling weight and provide a safer and healthy way to diet.

Recipes with certain foods are identified to slow down aging primarily because of their high nucleic acid content, as discussed in Chapter 6. Try to include recipes with the following foods as a part of your daily meal: asparagus, mushrooms, beets, collard greens, cauliflower, spinach, soybean sprouts.

Appropriate combinations of foods are provided by the menus in Appendixes B and C. Combinations of certain Eastern foods, unfamiliar to many Westerners, are provided along with a recipe in Appendix A.

SOUPS

Italian Vegetable Soup*

  1¼ cups chopped onions
  ½ cup chopped celery
  ½ cup chopped carrots
  1¾ cups chopped turnips
  2 cups diced zucchini
  3 sliced mushrooms
  ½ cup sliced greenbeans
  2 28-ounce canned diced tomatoes
  ½ 15-ounce canned tomato paste
  4 cups water

Sources Consulted for Recipes: Zurbel, R. and Zurbel, V. *The Vegetarian Family*, Prentice-Hall, Inc. (1978). *Time-Life Books on cooking of Italy and India* (1978, 1972). Doyle, R. *The Vegetarian Handbook*, Crown Publishers, Inc. (1979). Singh, B. *Mrs. Balbir Singh's Indian Cookery*, 6th ed., Mills and Boon Ltd., London (1971). Pritikin, N. *The Pritikin Program for Diet and Exercise*, Grosset and Dunlop, Inc. (1979). Frank, B. S. *Dr. Frank's No-Aging Diet*, The Dial Press (1976). Lin, F. *Florence Lin's Chinese Vegetarian Cookbook*, Hawthorn Books, Inc. (1976).

    2 bay leaves
    ½ teaspoon onion powder
    ½ teaspoon garlic powder
    ½ teaspoon Italian seasoning
    1 teaspoon dried parsley

Heat the water and the tomato products to a boil. Add all the vegetables except zucchini. Bring to a boil once again, turn down heat and simmer until vegetables are half done. Add the zucchini and the seasonings. Continue cooking until done.

    Makes about 16 servings

Tomato-Vegetable Soup*

    1 cup chopped onion
    1 cup chopped celery
    1 cup chopped carrots
    ½ cup chopped green pepper
    1 cup shredded white cabbage
    ⅓ cup diced potato
    ½ cup frozen 'mixed' vegetables
    7 cups water
    1 cup canned tomato juice
    1 cup canned diced tomatoes
    2 tablespoons lemon juice
    ¼ teaspoon marjoram
    ¼ teaspoon basil
    ½ teaspoon onion powder
    ½ teaspoon garlic powder
    ½ teaspoon dried parsley

Bring the water and tomato products to a boil. Add all the vegetables and the seasonings. Reduce heat and simmer until the vegetables are tender.

    Serves 8

Beet Borscht or Beet Soup*

    15 young, small beets
    1 16-ounce canned sauerkraut
    1 16-ounce canned tomato juice
    2 teaspoons lemon juice
    2 teaspoons vinegar
    Dash of allspice
    Dash of cloves
    Water as required

Scrub the beets clean and boil them until they are done. Run them under cold water and remove the skins. Dice the beets and add with the other ingredients to a soup pot. Bring the soup to a boil, then simmer it slowly until the flavors are well blended (about 25 minutes), adding water as needed to maintain desired consistency.

Serve hot or cold. Pass a bowl of chopped green onions as additional garnish.
Serves 8 to 10

This recipe is suggested to slow down aging.

Tomato-Okra Soup*

    1 7-ounce package frozen Chinese pea pods
    2 cups shredded green cabbage
    2 cups chopped mixed vegetables (carrots, celery, onion, or others of your choice),
        fresh or frozen
    3 cups canned tomato juice
    $\frac{1}{2}$ teaspoon cumin or other desired seasoning
    3 cups water
    1 7-ounce package frozen chopped okra

Bring water and tomato juice to a boil. Add all the ingredients, except the okra. Reduce heat and gently simmer the soup for about an hour. Add the okra during the last 10 to 15 minutes of the cooking period. Add more water if a thinner soup is desired. Serve hot.

Makes 6 to 8 servings

Southern Vegetable Soup*

    $\frac{1}{2}$ cup diced turnips
    $\frac{1}{2}$ cup diced rutabagas
    $\frac{1}{2}$ cup chopped onions
    $\frac{1}{3}$ cup chopped carrots
    $\frac{1}{3}$ cup cauliflower buds
    $\frac{1}{2}$ cup chopped broccoli
    $\frac{1}{3}$ cup halved brussels sprouts
    $\frac{1}{3}$ cup chopped tomatoes
    $\frac{1}{4}$ small head cabbage, shredded
    $\frac{1}{4}$ cup chopped summer squash (zucchini, crookneck, or scalloped)
    $\frac{1}{4}$ cup chopped mustard greens (optional)
    $\frac{1}{4}$ to $\frac{1}{2}$ teaspoon each oregano, basil, and garlic powder
    1 teaspoon grated sapsago (green cheese containing dried leaf of an aromatic legume,
        Trigonella coerulae) cheese (optional)
    8 cups water (approximate)

Bring about 2 cups of water to boil in the bottom of soup pot and add the root vegetables—turnips, rutabagas, onions, and carrots. Cook for a few minutes, adding more water as required to keep vegetables almost covered, until vegetables are partly done. Add the other vegetables to the soup pot and cover with water. Bring to a boil, then turn heat down to a simmer. Add oregano, basil, and garlic powder and continue cooking until vegetables are tender. If sapsago cheese is used,

add when soup is finished cooking. Add additional water if thinner soup is desired.
  Serves 10

Special Vegetable Soup*

  $\frac{1}{2}$ cup frozen lima beans
  $\frac{1}{2}$ cup frozen corn
  $\frac{1}{2}$ cup frozen green beans
  $\frac{3}{4}$ cup chopped carrots
  $\frac{3}{4}$ cup chopped celery
  $\frac{3}{4}$ cup chopped onions
  $\frac{3}{4}$ cup chopped potatoes
  $\frac{3}{4}$ cup chopped broccoli
  $\frac{3}{4}$ cup crookneck squash
  $\frac{3}{4}$ cup cauliflower florets
  $\frac{3}{4}$ cup sliced mushrooms
  $1\frac{1}{2}$ cups canned diced tomatoes
  $1\frac{1}{2}$ cups canned crushed tomatoes or tomato purée
  10 cups water
  2 bay leaves
  $\frac{1}{2}$ teaspoon oregano
  $\frac{1}{4}$ teaspoon dill seed
  1 teaspoon celery seed
  $\frac{1}{2}$ teaspoon marjoram
  $\frac{1}{4}$ teaspoon cumin (optional)
  1 teaspoon garlic powder
  1 teaspoon onion powder
  $\frac{1}{2}$ teaspoon Italian seasoning

Bring the water and the tomato products to a boil. Add all the vegetables except the squash. Reduce heat. Simmer until vegetables are almost done, then add the squash and the seasonings. Cook until done.
  Makes about 16 servings

Thick Vegetables Soup

  $\frac{1}{2}$ pound dry pinto beans
  $\frac{1}{2}$ pound dry lentils
  5 potatoes, diced
  $1\frac{1}{4}$ cups carrots, chopped
  $\frac{1}{2}$ pound dry barley
  $\frac{1}{2}$ bunch parsley, chopped (4 tablespoons)
  3 medium onions
  $\frac{1}{4}$ cup oil
  1 tablespoon soy sauce
  5 small tomatoes (canned if not in season)
  $\frac{1}{2}$ gallon can green beans
  Seasonings (to taste)

Soak the pinto beans and lentils overnight in water to cover. Drain. Cook the beans and lentils in fresh water until they are almost done. Add the potatoes, carrots, barley, parsley, and onions and cook until vegetables are tender. Add other ingredients at the end of cooking. Simmer to blend flavor. Add other seasonings to taste (e.g., Kitchen Bouquet, pepper, garlic, Royal soup flavorings).

Makes 15 servings of 1¼ cups each

Split Pea Soup

> **2 cups dried split peas**
> **2 quarts water**
> **1 onion, finely diced**
> **2 whole carrots, scraped**
> **2 sprigs (shoots) parsley, diced**
> **2 celery stalks**
> **¼ teaspoon pepper**
> **1 bay leaf**

Soak the peas in water overnight. Drain. Place them in a large soup pot with water; add the remaining ingredients. Bring to a boil, then reduce heat, and cover. Simmer for 2 hours, or until the peas have disintegrated. Rub all the soup through a food mill into another pot, or blend it until the mixture is reduced to a smooth soup.

Serves 8

Lima Bean Soup

> **1½ cups dried lima beans (or 3 cups frozen lima beans)**
> **1½ cups chopped celery**
> **1½ cups chopped carrots**
> **1½ cups chopped onions**
> **½ cup finely chopped green pepper**
> **1½ cups green beans, cut into 2-inch lengths, or frozen cut green beans**
> **2 to 3 tomatoes, chopped into small chunks, skin and all**
> **Water as required**
> **Suggested seasonings: bay leaf, basil, black pepper, and vinegar to taste**

Rinse and soak the beans overnight or for several hours in enough water to cover. Drain. Re-cover them with water to about 3 inches above the surface of the beans. You can also use 3 cups frozen lima beans instead of the dried. Simply cook the frozen beans for several minutes before adding the other ingredients. Add the bay leaf, and cook until the beans are tender. Replenish the water in the bean pot to about 3 inches above the bean surface. Add the celery, carrots, onions, green pepper, and green beans. (If frozen green beans are used, add them about 10 minutes later.) Add more water as required to keep the soup at desired consistency and to prevent any sticking. Toward the end of the cooking period, when the vegetables are almost tender, remove about 1/3 of the soup and blend it in a blender. Return the blended portion to the original soup pot and mix well. Serve hot.

Serves 6 to 8

Escarole Lentil Soup

2 cups dried lentils
1 quart water
1 onion diced
1 bay leaf
¼ teaspoon ground pepper
1 teaspoon paprika
1 head escarole

Pick over and wash the lentils. Soak them in water for several hours. Drain. Bring the water to a boil; add the lentils, onion, bay leaf, pepper, and paprika. Cook the lentil mixture over a very low heat, stirring occasionally, until the lentils are soft, about 1½ to 2 hours. Meanwhile, wash the escarole and trim off all of the white parts, using only the green leaves. Place the escarole in a saucepan, cover with water, and cook until soft. Drain. Add the escarole to the lentil soup just before it is ready to serve. The lentils should be soft but about half will retain their shape.

Serves 6

This recipe is suggested to slow down aging.

SALADS AND YOGURT DISHES

Salads are generally low in calories unless high calorie dressing is used. These are valuable for minerals, vitamins and cellulose. Yogurt dishes (*Raytas*) that always have a yogurt base, are mixed with fruits, vegetables, and seasonings (for low calories, make yogurt from skim or low-fat milk). These are frequently served with Indian meals, and like a salad, provide a cooling contrast to the main highly seasoned dishes of a meal.

Raw Mushroom Salad (*Insalata di Funghi Crudi*)

½ pound fresh mushrooms, thinly sliced
2 teaspoons lemon juice
¼ cup thinly sliced scallion greens
3 tablespoons olive oil
½ teaspoon salt

In a serving bowl, toss the mushrooms with the lemon juice until the slices are lightly moistened. Then add the scallion greens, oil and salt and toss again. Chill the salad before serving it.

Serves 4

Italian Tomato Salad (*Insalata di Pomodori*)

> 5 medium-sized firm ripe tomatoes, sliced ¼ inch thick
> ½ cup olive oil
> 2 tablespoons wine vinegar or lemon juice
> 1 tablespoon finely cut fresh basil or 1 teaspoon dried basil
> ¼ teaspoon finely chopped garlic
> 1 teaspoon salt
> Freshly ground black pepper
> 2 tablespoons thinly sliced scallions
> 1 tablespoon finely chopped fresh parsley

Arrange the tomato slices in slightly overlapping concentric circles on a deep round plate or platter. For the dressing, thoroughly mix the oil, vinegar, basil, garlic, salt and a few grindings of pepper and spoon or pour this over the tomatoes. Combine the scallions and parsley and sprinkle the mixture evenly on top.

    Serves 4 to 6

Indian Mixed Vegetable Salad (*Salaad*)

> 2 large onions, peeled, cut in half lengthwise, then cut lengthwise into paper-thin slivers
> 2 large firm, ripe tomatoes, washed, stemmed and cut crosswise into ¼-inch thick slices
> 24 radishes, trimmed and washed
> 2 medium-sized lemons, each cut lengthwise in quarters
> 3 fresh hot green peppers, each about 3 inches long, washed, slit in half lengthwise and seeded
> ¼ cup fresh lemon juice
> 1 teaspoon salt
> Freshly ground black pepper

Spread the slivers of onion evenly over the entire surface of a large serving platter and arrange the tomato slices in a ring around the edge. Arrange the radishes, lemon wedges and hot green peppers decoratively around the tomatoes, and sprinkle the vegetables evenly with the lemon juice, salt and a liberal grinding of black pepper.

    Serves 4 to 6

Indian Tomato, Onion and Ginger Salad (*Cachumbar*)

> 2 medium-sized tomatoes, washed, stemmed and coarsely chopped
> ¼ cup finely chopped onions
> ¼ cup coarsely chopped fresh coriander
> 3 tablespoons fresh lemon juice
> 1 tablespoon scraped, finely slivered fresh ginger root
> 1 teaspoon salt
> 2 fresh hot green peppers, each about 3 inches long, washed, stemmed, seeded and cut crosswise into thin slices

In a small serving bowl, combine the tomatoes, onions, coriander, lemon juice, ginger root and salt, and turn them about with a spoon to mix them thoroughly. Sprinkle the top with hot green peppers, and refrigerate for at least 1 hour, or until thoroughly chilled.

Serves 3 to 4

Indian Tomato, Onion and Beet Salad (*Tamatar Salaad*)

> 3 tablespoons vegetable oil (optional)
> 2 tablespoon fresh lemon juice
> 1 tablespoon finely chopped fresh mint
> 1 tablespoon finely chopped fresh coriander
> 1 teaspoon salt
> 2 large onions, peeled and each cut crosswise into 6 slices
> 2 large uncooked beets, preferably white beets, peeled and each cut crosswise into 6 thin slices
> 2 large firm, ripe tomatoes, washed, stemmed, and each cut crosswise into 6 slices
> 2 fresh hot green peppers washed, stemmed, and cut crosswise into thin rounds

Combine the vegetable oil, lemon juice, mint, coriander and salt in a bowl, and stir with a fork or a whisk until the ingredients are thoroughly blended.

Stack the onions, beets and tomatoes in the following fashion: Arrange 6 of the onion slices side by side on a large serving platter and place a beet and tomato slice on top of each. Cover each stack with another layer of onions, beets and tomatoes. Sprinkle the peppers over the stacks, and sprinkle their tops evenly with the oil-and-lemon dressing. Marinate at room temperature for 30 minutes or in the refrigerator for at least 1 hour before serving.

Serves 6

Greek Salad

> 3 cups raw spinach or lettuce (or combine)
> 2 tomatoes, quartered
> 1 cup fresh, black pitted olives
> 1 pound crumbled or diced feta cheese
> 3 stalks celery diced

Combine all ingredients in a bowl and serve with lemon juice or your favorite dressing.

Serves about 8

Spinach Salad with Sesame Seed Dressing

> 1 pound spinach leaves
> 1 cup sunflower seeds or 1 cup chopped walnuts
> 1 bunch parsley, chopped fine
> $\frac{1}{2}$ cup safflower oil
> $\frac{1}{2}$ cup lemon juice
> 1 tablespoon honey

4 tablespoons sesame seeds
$\frac{1}{4}$ teaspoon cayenne
$\frac{1}{2}$ teaspoon sea salt

Combine spinach leaves with seeds or nuts and parsley. Blend remaining ingredients until smooth and pour over salad as desired.

Serves 4 to 6

Spinach and Mushroom Salad

1 pound fresh spinach
$\frac{1}{4}$ pound fresh mushrooms
1 hard-boiled egg white
$\frac{1}{4}$ cup tarragon vinegar
2 tablespoons water
$\frac{1}{8}$ teaspoon ground pepper
$\frac{1}{8}$ teaspoon ground paprika
1 tablespoon undiluted frozen orange juice concentrate, thawed

Trim and wash the spinach carefully and place in a salad bowl. Wash and slice the mushrooms; add them to the spinach. Discard the yolk of the egg, and chop the white; add it to the spinach. Combine the vinegar, water, pepper, paprika and orange juice; pour the dressing over the salad. Toss and serve.

Serves 4 to 6

This recipe is suggested to slow down aging.

Bamboo Salad

1 cup bamboo shoots
1 cup bean sprouts
$\frac{1}{2}$ cup water chestnuts, chopped
$\frac{1}{2}$ cup celery diced
$\frac{3}{4}$ cup string beans, chopped
1 cup watercress, chopped
1 tablespoon sesame seeds

In bowl, combine ingredients. Serve with or without a dressing.

Cole Slaw

$1\frac{1}{2}$ cups chopped green onions
$2\frac{1}{2}$ cups shredded red cabbage
6 cups shredded green cabbage
1 cup finely chopped dill pickles
1 cup chopped red pepper
3 cups grated carrots
2 cups peeled apple slices
$\frac{1}{2}$ cup undiluted frozen apple juice concentrate, thawed
$\frac{1}{4}$ cup apple cider vinegar or lemon juice

      1 teaspoon ground ginger
      ¼ teaspoon garlic powder
      1 tablespoon celery seed
      1 teaspoon dry mustard

Chop and shred the vegetables and pickles as desired. Place the apple slices in a blender together with the apple juice, vinegar, and spices; blend thoroughly. Pour the mixture over the chopped and shredded vegetables, mixing well. Refrigerate the cole slaw for several hours or overnight to blend the flavors. Serve chilled.

   Makes about 1 gallon or 16 of 8 oz servings

Herbed Chick-pea Salad

      1 cup chick-peas, cooked, but firm
      ½ cucumber, sliced
      ¼ cup fresh mint, chopped
      5 cups Chinese lettuce or iceberg lettuce, chopped and crispy
      2 tablespoons shelled sunflower seeds
      1 tablespoon parsley flakes
      2 teaspoons dill

In bowl, combine ingredients.

Soybean Salad

      1 can or 1 cup cooked soybeans; mayonnaise to taste
      1 stalk celery, finely chopped
      1 teaspoon celery seed
      Spike, Vegesalt, or sea salt to taste

Mix all ingredients and serve on salad platter. Or mash and serve on sandwiches like tuna salad. Add grated carrots if you like. Or add alfalfa sprouts for a chewy salad.

   Also try Chick-pea Salad, replacing soybeans with chick-peas in the above soybean recipe.

Mixed Bean Salad

      1 cup cooked garbanzos (chick-peas) (½ cup dry)
      1 cup cooked kidney beans (½ cup dry)
      1 cup cooked black beans (½ cup dry)
      1 cup cooked string beans
      ¼ cup diced pimiento
      ¼ cup diced onion
      2 tablespoons oil
      1 tablespoon lemon juice
      ¼ teaspoon salt
      ¼ teaspoon dried basil
      Dark leafy greens

Cook the garbanzos, kidnery beans, and black beans separately until they are tender but still firm. Drain well. Combine the beans with the rest of the ingredients except the greens. Toss well and refrigerate. Serve on bed of leafy greens.

Serves 4 to 6

SPROUTS

To sprout the seeds you need a wide-mouthed quart glass bottle, preferably a mason jar with a removable inner metal top and three grades of nylon mesh (available in fabric stores), extra fine, fine and medium; or wire mesh; or cheesecloth. You can also buy a ready-made sprouting kit at your health food store.

Place the seeds in jar and fill with water to soak overnight. Use 2 tablespoons of alfalfa seed, 6 of mung beans. The following morning place the fine mesh over the top of the jar, securing it in place with the open mason top or a rubber band. Drain off the soak water and fill with fresh water, then drain again. Place the jar on its side, spreading seeds out, and keep in a warm, dark corner. Rinse every morning and evening. As the sprouts grow and throw off the seeds hulls, change to a larger-screen top so you can rinse hulls away. With alfalfa seeds you can probably stay with a fine screen, but for the mung beans you will need a coarser screen to let the hulls get through. Sprouts develop in 3 to 5 days. When the first young leaves appear, place in direct sunlight for the development of chlorophyll. (Sprouts will become greener.) Wait about 8 hours after the last rinsing before refrigerating in a closed container.

The alfalfa seed is one of the easiest and best seeds to sprout. It is one of the most complete and nutritionally rich foods. In addition to its high potency of vitamins and minerals, it is high in protein. And alfalfa sprouts are delicious. These can be used in salads and on sandwiches in place of lettuce.

Sprouted mixtures of alfalfa, mung beans, and lentils are available in some health food store, or you can make your own. They make an excellent combination. Mung bean sprouts are a bit tough to eat raw, and you may steam or stir-fry them, in the wok. Among the other seeds and beans that can be sprouted are soybeans, barley, buckwheat, fava, lima, pinto, corn, cress clover, caraway, celery, dill, flax, fenugreek, garbanzos, kale, lettuce, millet, parsley, pumpkin, oats, sunflower, safflower, and wheat.

Wheat grass sprouts have been getting a lot of recognition for healing properties. The Hippocrates Health Center in Boston has treated cancer and other diseases with wheat grass therapy.

Sprout Salad

> **2 cups bean sprouts**
> **2 cups alfalfa sprouts**
> **1 cup raw mushrooms, sliced vertically**
> **$\frac{1}{2}$ cup chopped walnuts**

Combine ingredients and serve with Avocado Dressing. (see next salad dressings section for Avocado Dressing.)

This recipe is suggested to slow down aging.

Sprout Salad in Yogurt

> 1 cup mung bean sprouts
> 1 cup alfalfa sprouts
> 1 cup diced cucumber
> ½ cup chopped walnuts
> 4 cups yogurt

Mix all ingredients. Season to taste with sea salt and kelp. Or sweeten with honey.

Yogurt with Mint and Onion (*Pudine ka Rayta*)

> 3 tablespoons finely cut fresh mint
> 3 tablespoons finely chopped onions
> ½ teaspoon finely chopped fresh hot red or green pepper
> ½ teaspoon salt
> ⅛ teaspoon ground hot red pepper
> 1 cup unflavored yogurt

In a small serving bowl, combine the mint, onions, pepper, salt and red pepper. When they are thoroughly blended, stir in the yogurt. Taste for seasoning, cover tightly, and refrigerate for at least 1 hour, or until completely chilled. Before serving, decorate the rayta, if you like, with fresh whole mint leaves.

Serves 3 to 4

Variation: Finely chopped fresh tomatoes in place or/in addition to mint can be used. If red pepper is too hot, use black pepper instead.

Yogurt with Cucumber and Tomato (*Kheera ka Rayta*)

> 1 medium-sized cucumber
> 1 tablespoon finely chopped onions
> 1 tablespoon salt
> 1 small, firm ripe tomato, cut crosswise into ½-inch-thick rounds, sliced into ½-inch-wide strips and then into ½-inch cubes
> 1 tablespoon finely chopped fresh coriander
> 1 cup unflavored yogurt
> 1 teaspoon ground cumin, toasted in a small ungreased skillet over low heat for 30 seconds (optional)

With a small, sharp knife, peel the cucumber and slice it lengthwise into halves. Scoop out the seeds by running the tip of a teaspoon down the center of each half. Cut the cucumber lengthwise into 1/8-inch-thick slices, then crosswise into ½-inch pieces.

Combine the cucumber, onions and salt in a small bowl, and mix them together thoroughly with a spoon. Let the mixture rest at room temperature for 5 minutes or so, then squeeze the cucumbers gently between your fingers to remove the excess liquid.

Drop the cucumber pieces into a deep bowl, add the tomato and coriander, and toss them together gently but thoroughly. Combine the yogurt and cumin and put it over the vegetables, turning them about with a spoon to coat them evenly. Taste for seasoning, cover tightly, and refrigerate for at least 1 hour, or until completely chilled, before serving.

Serves 4

Yogurt with Spiced Potatoes (*Alu ka Rayta*)

>3 medium-sized firm boiling-type potatoes
>   (about 1 pound), scrubbed but not peeled
>2 tablespoons vegetable oil
>1 teaspoon black mustard seeds
>1 teaspoon cumin seeds
>3 tablespoons finely chopped onions
>1 teaspoon finely chopped fresh hot red or green pepper
>1 tablespoon finely chopped fresh coriander
>$\frac{1}{2}$ teaspoon salt
>1 cup unflavored yogurt

Drop the potatoes into enough boiling water to cover them completely and boil briskly, uncovered, until they are tender but still show some resistance when pierced with the point of a small, sharp knife. Drain the potatoes in a colander, peel and cut them into $\frac{1}{2}$-inch cubes.

In a heavy skillet, heat the vegetable oil over high heat until it starts to smoke. Stir in the mustard and cumin seeds and, when they crackle and begin to burst, immediately add the onions. Stirring constantly, add the pepper, coriander and potatoes.

Cook over moderate heat, turning the potatoes frequently with a spoon, until the cubes are well coated with the spice mixture. Remove the skillet from the heat and stir in the salt.

Place the yogurt in a small serving bowl, add the entire contents of the skillet, and toss gently together. Taste for seasoning, cover tightly, and refrigerate for at least 1 hour, or until completely chilled.

Serves 4 to 6

YOGURT WITH MINIATURE DEEP-FRIED CHICK-PEA FLOUR BALLS (PAKORA KA RAYTA)

Chick-Pea Balls (*Pakora*)

>$\frac{1}{2}$ cup chick-pea flour (*besan*)
>$\frac{1}{2}$ teaspoon salt

¼ cup cold water
2 cups vegetable oil for deep frying

In a deep bowl make a smooth, thin batter of ½ cup of chick-pea flour, ½ teaspoon of salt and the water, stirring them together with a spoon or with your fingers.

Pour 2 cups of vegetable oil into a heavy skillet or wok, or pour oil into a deep fryer to a depth of 2 to 3 inches, and heat.

To shape the *pakoras*, hold a hand grater with openings ¼ inch in diameter above the deep fryer, then pick up a little of the batter with your fingers and press it through the grater into the hot oil. In 30 seconds, or as soon as the *pakoras* are brown, remove them from the oil with a slotted spoon and transfer them to paper towels to drain.

Repeat this process until all the batter is fried. (There should be about 3/4 cup of *pakoras*.) Cool the *pakoras* to room temperature before using them.

Yogurt

    1 cup unflavored yogurt, chilled
    1 teaspoon ground cumin
    ½ teaspoon salt
    ¼ teaspoon ground hot red pepper
    2 tablespoons finely chopped fresh coriander

Just before serving, stir the yogurt, cumin and ½ teaspoon of salt together in a small serving bowl. Gently fold half of the *pakoras* into the yogurt mixture, and spread the rest of them on top. Sprinkle with red pepper and coriander.

Serves 4 to 6

SALAD DRESSINGS AND CHUTNEYS

Herb Vinegar Dressing

    1 cup wine vinegar
    ¼ cup fresh dill (or ½ teaspoon dried dillweed)
    ¼ cup snipped fresh chives
    ⅓ cup snipped fresh mint
    1 clove garlic, finely chopped

Combine all the ingredients. Let the dressing stay in the refrigerator for at least 4 days (to get maximum flavor). Strain to remove herbs.

Makes about 1¼ cups

French Dressing

    1 onion, chopped
    1 cucumber, chopped

½ green pepper, chopped (optional)
2 cups water
2 cups vinegar (cider, wine, or rice vinegar) juice of 2 lemons and some of the pulp
½ teaspoon garlic powder
½ teaspoon ground black pepper
1 teaspoon ground celery seed
1 teaspoon dillweed
3 teaspoons chopped parsley

In a blender, grate the chopped onion, cucumber, and green pepper, if used, together with water. Add the other ingredients; continue blending until all is well blended. Chill and serve.

To make Tomato French Dressing, substitute tomato juice for part of the water in the above recipe.

Makes about 5½ cups

Italian Dressing

¼ cup lemon juice
¼ cup cider vinegar
¼ cup apple juice, unsweetened
½ teaspoon oregano
½ teaspoon dry mustard
½ teaspoon onion powder
½ teaspoon garlic powder
½ teaspoon paprika
⅛ teaspoon thyme
⅛ teaspoon rosemary

Combine all the ingredients in a blender. Blend well. Chill and refrigerate overnight or better yet, two days—to permit flavors to blend.

Makes about 3/4 cup

Russian Dressing

¾ cup cider or rice vinegar
¾ cup water
⅛ cup lemon juice
¼ medium onion, chopped
1 tablespoon garlic powder
Dash of white pepper
Dash of paprika
2 small carrots, grated

Blend all ingredients, except carrots, in blender, until well mixed. Float grated carrots in dressing. Chill before serving.

Makes about 2 cups

Avocado Dressing

> 2 avocados, peeled and mashed
> 1 tomato, skinned and sliced
> ½ cup lemon juice
> 1 tablespoon honey (optional)
> Spices and seasonings to your own taste

Blend ingredients until smooth.

Tomato-Lemon Dressing

> ¾ cup canned tomato juice
> ¼ cup lemon juice
> ¼ cup unsweetened apple juice
> ⅓ cup chopped celery
> 1½ cups chopped onion
> ½ clove garlic, minced

Combine all the ingredients in a blender and blend well. Chill and serve.
Makes about 3½ cups

Fresh Mango Chutney with Hot Pepper (*Corom Chatni*)

> 1 medium-sized firm but underripe mango (about 1 pound)
> 1 fresh hot green pepper, stemmed, slit in half lengthwise, seeded and cut crosswise
>   into thin rings
> 1 tablespoon finely chopped fresh coriander
> 1 tablespoon salt
> ⅛ teaspoon ground hot red pepper

Wash the mango under cold running water and dry it with paper towels. Without removing the skin, cut the flesh of the mango away from the large seed inside. Discard the seed and cut the flesh of the mango into paper-thin slices.

Place the mango in a serving bowl, add the green pepper, coriander, salt and red pepper, and toss gently with a spoon until the ingredients are thoroughly mixed. Let the chutney marinate in the refrigerator for 1 to 2 hours before serving. (Tightly covered and refrigerated, it can be kept for 1 day.)
Makes about 1 cup

Fresh Ginger Chutney (*Adrak Chatni*)

> ½ cup fresh lemon juice
> 1 cup scraped, coarsely chopped fresh ginger root
> ½ cup white raisins
> 2 tablespoons finely chopped garlic
> 2 teaspoons salt

Combine the lemon juice, ginger, raisins, garlic and salt, and blend at high speed for 30 seconds. Turn the machine off and scrape down the sides of the jar with a rubber spatula, then blend again for 30 seconds longer, or until the mixture is reduced to a smooth purée.

Serve the chutney at once or cover tightly and refrigerate until ready to use. It may be kept in the refrigerator for 1 to 2 days.

Makes about 1½ cups

Fresh Coriander Chutney (*Dhanya Chatni*)

¼ cup fresh lemon juice
¼ cup water
¼ pound fresh coriander stems and leaves thoroughly washed and coarsely chopped, about 2 cups tightly packed
¼ cup peeled, finely chopped fresh coconut
¼ cup finely chopped onions
2 tablespoons scraped, finely chopped fresh ginger root
2 teaspoons chopped fresh hot green pepper
1 teaspoon sugar
1 teaspoon salt
¼ teaspoon freshly ground black pepper

Combine the lemon juice, water and ½ cup of the coriander, and blend at high speed for 30 seconds, or until the mixture is reduced to a purée. Turn the machine off and scrape down the sides of the jar with a rubber spatula. Then add another ½ cup of coriander, blend for 30 seconds, and stop the machine again. Repeat until all of the coriander has been puréed.

Add the coconut, onions, ginger, green pepper, sugar, salt and black pepper, and blend again. When the mixture is perfectly smooth, taste and add more sugar or salt if desired.

Serve immediately. If the chutney is not to be used at once, cover it tightly and refrigerate it. (The chutney may be kept in the refrigerator for about 1 week.)

Makes about 2 cups

Cooked Tomato Chutney (*Tamatar Chatni*)

3 medium-sized firm, ripe tomatoes (about 1 pound), washed, cored and coarsely chopped
1 cup malt vinegar
1 cup finely chopped onions
1 1-inch piece of cinnamon stick
1 tablespoon salt
1 cup imported Indian jaggery, coarsely crumbled, or substitute 1 cup dark-brown sugar combined with 1 tablespoon dark molasses (optional)
2 tablespoons scraped, finely chopped fresh ginger root
1 tablespoon finely chopped garlic
8 whole cloves
½ teaspoon chopped fresh hot red or green pepper
¼ cup finely chopped fresh coriander leaves and stems

$\frac{1}{2}$ **cup mustard oil, or substitute 3 tablespoons vegetable oil (optional)**
2 tablespoons black mustard seeds (optional)

In a heavy 2- to 3-quart enameled or stainless-steel saucepan, combine the tomatoes, vinegar, onions, cinnamon and salt. Stirring constantly, bring to a boil over
moderate heat. Stir in the jaggery (or brown sugar and molasses), then add the
ginger, garlic, cloves, pepper and coriander. Still stirring, cook over moderate
heat for 5 minutes.

Heat the mustard oil in a small skillet until it begins to smoke, stir in the
mustard seeds, and as soon as they begin to splutter add them, oil and all, to the
tomato mixture. Stirring frequently, boil briskly for 8 to 10 minutes, until the
chutney begins to thicken. Cool to room temperature before serving.

Covered tightly and refrigerated, *tamatear chatni* may be safely kept for 3 or 4
weeks.

Makes about $1\frac{1}{2}$ cups

Fresh Mint Chutney (*Pudina Chatni*)

$\frac{1}{4}$ **cup malt vinegar**
2 tablespoons water
2 cups fresh mint leaves, thoroughly washed and tightly packed
1 fresh hot red or green pepper, about 3 inches long, stemmed, seeded and chopped
2 tablespoons finely chopped onions
1 teaspoon salt

Combine the vinegar, water and $\frac{1}{2}$ cup of the mint leaves, and blend at high speed
for 30 seconds, or until the mixture is reduced to a smooth purée. Turn the machine off and scrape down the sides of the jar with a rubber spatula. Then add
another $\frac{1}{2}$ cup of mint, blend for 30 seconds, and stop the machine again. Repeat
until all of the mint has been puréed, then add the pepper, onions and salt, and
blend again. Serve at once. If the chutney is not to be used at once, cover tightly
and refrigerate. It may be kept in the refrigerator for 1 or 2 days.

Makes about 1 cup

Tamarind Chutney (*Imli Chatni*)

$\frac{1}{4}$ **cup tightly packed dried tamarind pulp (about 2 ounces)**
1 cup boiling water
1 tablespoon scraped, finely chopped fresh ginger root
1 tablespoon fresh lemon juice
1 teaspoon crumbled imported Indian jaggery, or substitute dark-brown sugar
  combined with dark molasses (optional)
1 teaspoon salt
2 tablespoons finely chopped fresh coriander

Place the tamarind pulp in a small bowl and pour the boiling water over it.
Stirring and mashing occasionally with a spoon, let the tamarind soak for 1 hour,
or until the pulp separates and dissolves in the water. Rub the tamarind through a

fine sieve set over a bowl, pressing down hard with the back of a spoon before discarding the seeds and fibers. Or purée it through a food mill.

Add the ginger, lemon juice, jaggery (or brown sugar and molasses) and the salt to the purée, and stir together vigorously. Taste for seasoning. Serve at once or cover tightly and store in the refrigerator for up to 2 days.

Just before serving, pour the chutney into a small bowl and sprinkle the top with coriander.

Makes about 1 cup

VEGETABLES

Stuffed Mushrooms

Recipe No. 1

> 20 medium mushrooms, washed
> ½ cup bean curd, mashed
> ½ medium onion, peeled and minced
> 2 stalks celery, minced
> 1 vegetable bouillion cube
> 2 teaspoons cornstarch or 1 teaspoon arrowroot
> ¾ cup warm water

Remove stems from mushrooms. Chop stems. In bowl, combine stems with bean curd, onion and celery. Stuff mixture into mushroom caps. Arrange stuffed mushrooms in frying pan. In cup, dissolve bouillion cube and cornstarch in water. Pour into pan. Cover. Cook over low heat for 15 minutes.

Recipe No. 2

> 12 large mushrooms
> 1 tablespoon chopped parsley
> ¼ teaspoon garlic powder
> ¼ teaspoon onion powder
> 2 tablespoons permissible bread crumbs
> 1 egg white

Remove the stems from the mushrooms; trim the ends and chop stems fine. Add the parsley, garlic powder, onion powder, and bread crumbs. Beat the egg white with a fork until it is frothy and mix with the chopped mushrooms. Spoon the egg-white mixture into the mushroom caps. Place the mushrooms in a nonstick baking pan and bake in a 400° F. (205°C.) oven for 20 minutes.

Serves 4

Mushroom recipes are suggested to slow down aging.

Stuffed Zucchini (*Zucchini Ripieni*)

> 3 large zucchini
> 1 onion, thinly sliced

1 green pepper diced
1 clove garlic, minced
½ cup chopped fresh tomatoes
1 cup tomato juice
1 teaspoon dried oregano
1 slice sourdough toast

Cut the zucchini in half lengthwise. Scoop out the pulp, leaving boatlike ¼-inch-thick shells. Save the zucchini shells for stuffing. Dice the scooped-out zucchini; place them in a large nonstick skillet with the onion, green pepper, garlic, chopped tomatoes, ¼ cup of the tomato juice , and oregano. Cook until the vegetables are limp. Fill the reserved zucchini shells with the cooked mixture and arrange in a baking dish. Pour the remaining tomato juice around the stuffed zucchini. Crumble the toast and sprinkle it on the tops of the stuffing. Bake in a 350 °F. (180°C.) oven for 30 minutes, or until the shells are tender.

Serve with tomato juice gravy spooned over the shells.

Serves 6

Asparagus with Lemon-Parsley Sauce

1 bunch fresh asparagus
¼ cup lemon juice
2 tablespoons chopped fresh parsley

Trim the scales and the woody ends from the asparagus. Wash well. Tie them loosely together in a bunch. Stand them upright in the bottom of a double boiler; and several inches of water and invert the top of the boiler to serve as a cover. (In this way the tender tops will steam while the bottoms boil.) Cook the asparagus just until they are tender. Remove them from the water, cut the string. Arrange on a platter. Stir the lemon juice and fresh parsley together; pour this over asparagus and serve.

Serves 4 to 6

This recipe is suggested to slow down aging.

Stir-Fried Asparagus (*Ch'ao Lou Sun*)

1 small bunch asparagus (about 1 pound)
2 tablespoons peanut or corn oil
1 teaspoon salt
½ teaspoon sugar
1 tablespoon water

Break off and discard the tough end of each asparagus spear. Soak the tender spears in lukewarm water for 15 minutes. With your fingers, pick off and discard the triangle leaves along the spear except for the tender ones at the top. Wash the asparagus thoroughly and drain well. Roll-cut the spears and set aside. You should have about 3 cups.

Heat a wok until hot. Add the oil, then the asparagus, and stir-fry over high heat for 2 minutes. Add the salt and sugar and sprinkle on the water. Stir and mix well for another 2 minutes. If the asparagus spears are not tender, add 1 more tablespoon of water, cover the pot, and simmer for 1 minute longer. Remove and serve hot.

Serves 4 when served with other dishes.

Variation: Zucchini may be used instead of asparagus. After cleaning, cut zucchini into 1-inch chunks. Cook in the same manner as the asparagus.

Chinese Braised Fresh Bean Curd (*Hung Shao Lao Tou Fu*)

6, 3 × 3 × ¾-inch (8 × 8 × 2 centimeters) squares fresh firm bean curd or 4,
   4 × 4 × 1½-inch (10 × 10 × 4 centimeters) squares fresh tender bean curd
Cold water
3 tablespoons peanut or corn oil
1 tablespoon finely shredded fresh ginger root
½ tablespoon sugar
3 tablespoons soy sauce
⅛ teaspoon monosodium glutamate
½ cup water

Put the bean curd in a saucepan and cover with cold water, 2 inches above the bean curd, slowly bring to a boil and cook over medium heat for 30 minutes. Let cool, then drain. Cut each bean curd piece into eighths and squeeze gently to remove excess water. Set aside near the cooking area.

Heat a saucepan over medium heat until hot. Add the oil, ginger root and cut-up bean curd. Gently stir-fry for 2 minutes. Add the sugar, soy sauce, monosodium glutamate, and ½ cup water. Cover and bring to a boil, then simmer over low heat for about 1 hour, basting 2 or 3 times. Serve hot. This dish can be reheated.

Serves 3 to 4 or up to 8 when served with other dishes

Note: ½ to 1 cup braised fresh mushrooms, including oil, sautéed fresh mushrooms, fresh or canned bamboo shoots, dried mushrooms, and/or flat-tip bamboo shoots (soaked until soft) may be added to the bean curd.

Chinese Vegetable Egg Fu Jung (*Fu Jung Tan*)

4 dried mushrooms
⅓ cup fresh or canned bamboo shoots, cut in julienne strips
½ cup soaked dried flat-tip bamboo shoots, cut in julienne strips
2 cups fresh bean sprouts, washed and drained
1 scallion, finely shredded
5 tablespoons peanut or corn oil
6 large eggs
1½ teaspoons salt
⅛ teaspoon white pepper

$^1\!/_4$ teaspoon monosodium glutamate
$^1\!/_2$ teaspoon sesame oil

Wash and soak the dried mushrooms in $^1\!/_2$ cup hot water until soft. Drain, remove the stems, and finely shred. Set aside on a plate with the bamboo shoots, flat-tip bamboo shoots, bean sprouts, and scallion.

Heat 2 tablespoons oil in wok over high heat. Stir-fry the scallion, bean sprouts, both kinds of bamboo shoots, and mushrooms for 2 minutes. Remove and let cool. Beat the eggs thoroughly. Add the vegetable mixture to the beaten eggs, then add salt, pepper, monosodium glutamate, and sesame oil. Mix well with the eggs.

Now, heat a wok until very hot. Add the remaining 3 tablespoons oil. Before the oil reaches the smoking point, pour in the egg mixture. Using a spatula, push the eggs back and forth, then flip and turn the eggs so that the pieces will be slightly brown on the outside yet soft inside. Serve hot.

Serves 4 for brunch or up to 6 when served with other dishes

Variations: Stir-fried fresh mushrooms or canned mushrooms may be used instead of dried mushrooms. Shredded celery, carrot or other vegetables may be used instead of dried bamboo shoots.

Chinese Spinach with Bean Curd Soup (*Po Ts'ai Tou Fu Keng*)

> 1 pound fresh spinach
> 3 tablespoons peanut or corn oil
> 1 teaspoon salt
> $^3\!/_4$ teaspoon sugar
> 1, $4 \times 4 \times 1^1\!/_2$-inch ($10 \times 10 \times 4$ centimeter) square fresh tender bean curd, cut up
> 3 cups water
> 2 tablespoons cornstarch combined with $^1\!/_4$ cup cold water; Sesame oil
> Salt to taste

Cut the spinach leaves, if too large, into pieces 2 inches long. Wash and drain thoroughly.

Heat a large wok until very hot, then add the peanut oil. Taking as much spinach as you can hold in both hands, cover the hot oil surface on the wok so that the oil does not spatter. Stir until the spinach is slightly wilted and then add the rest. Stir-fry until all of the spinach is wilted. Add the salt and sugar and stir to mix well. Use chopsticks or a fork to remove the spinach from the wok and place in a saucepan (discard the liquid in the wok). Add the spinach, bean curd, and water to the saucepan and bring to a boil. Mix the cornstarch and cold water, add, stirring well until soup thickens. Add a few drops sesame oil and salt to taste before serving.

Serves 6

Note: Fresh spinach, when sold loose by weight, is left uncut with roots intact. The stem of the leaf, which is attached to the plant, is pink. This pink part of the stem is sweet and has a good flavor. When the loose fresh spinach is cooked, it tastes far better than the prewashed spinach packed in cellophane bags. The pink stems of the spinach should be cut into 2-inch long pieces along with the leaves and split into 2 to 4 stalks for easy washing and serving.

Variations: Chinese leeks, chrysanthemum greens, and amaranth can be used instead of spinach. Also frozen spinach may be used instead of fresh spinach.

Harvard Beets

> 1 bunch fresh beets
> ¼ cup lemon juice
> 1 tablespoon vinegar
> 2 tablespoons undiluted frozen apple juice concentrate, thawed
> 2 tablespoons cornstarch

Trim and peel the beets. Place them in a saucepan, cover with water, and cook, covered, until the beets are tender. Slice the beets. Measure 1½ cups of beet liquid and return that to the saucepan; add the lemon juice, vinegar, and apple juice mixed with the cornstarch. Heat and stir until the mixture thickens and becomes clear. Return the sliced beets to the sauce and heat through.

> Serves 4 to 6

This recipe is suggested to slow down aging.

Basic Eggplant Curry

> 1 medium-size eggplant
> 2 medium onion, sliced
> ½ cup coconut or regular milk
> 1 teaspoon lemon juice
> 1 teaspoon ground mustard
> 1 teaspoon salt
> 1 teaspoon curry powder
> 2 tablespoons butter
> 3 teaspoons peanut or coconut oil
> 1 teaspoon chili powder (optional)
> ½ teaspoon fresh ginger, chopped (optional)

In pot, boil eggplant for 6 minutes. Then drain and dice. In frying pan, sauté onions, lemon juice, and spices in butter for 10 minutes. Add eggplant and sauté for another 5 minutes.

Add oil and milk, cover, and cook over low heat until most of the liquid is gone. Usually eaten with home-made Indian bread—*chapati* or *puri.*

Basic Vegetable Curry

> 4 tablespoons oil
> 2 teaspoons mustard seed
> 2 teaspoons turmeric

1 teaspoon coriander seed
1 teaspoon cayenne
2 teaspoons cumin seed
1 teaspoon salt
1 cup carrots, diced
2 cups string beans, cut
1 cup peas, fresh or frozen
1 cup potatoes, diced
2 cups water
$\frac{1}{2}$ cup yogurt

Heat oil in large pot. Add mustard seed until it dances; and remaining spices and salt, then stir. Add vegetables. Stir again and add water. Bring to a boil, add yogurt, stir and simmer for 20 minutes.

Ratatouille*

$\frac{1}{2}$ eggplant, peeled and cut into chunks
1 cup sliced zucchini
1 green pepper, cut into chunks
1 large onion, cut into chunks
2 stalks celery, cut in diagonal slices (Chinese style)
2 shallots, finely chopped (optional)
1 clove garlic, minced
2 to 3 tablespoons chopped fresh parsley
$\frac{1}{8}$ teaspoon ground pepper
2 cups fresh tomatoes, cut into chunks, or diced canned tomatoes

Combine all the ingredients (except the fresh tomatoes) in a large pot or skillet. Cover and cook over low heat for about 20 minutes. Uncover and cook 15 minutes more over moderate heat, stirring with a spoon to prevent scorching. Add the tomatoes until they become mushy. Serve hot.

This dish is easily varied by adding additional seasonings as desired, such as canned *salsa*, Italian seasoning, *oregano*, basil or any combination of the above.

Serves 8

Italian White Beans with Tomatoes and Garlic (*Fagioli all'Uccelletto*)

3 cups canned cannellini or other white beans ($1\frac{1}{2}$ one-pound cans); or $1\frac{1}{2}$ cups
    dry white kidney, marrow, great Northern or navy beans
$1\frac{1}{2}$ quarts water
$\frac{1}{4}$ cup olive oil
1 teaspoon finely chopped garlic
$\frac{1}{4}$ teaspoon sage leaves, crumbled
2 large ripe tomatoes, peeled, seeded, gently squeezed of excess juice, and
    coarsely chopped
$\frac{1}{2}$ teaspoon salt
Freshly ground black pepper
1 tablespoon wine vinegar

If you are using dry beans, combine them with the water in a 3- to 4-quart saucepan and bring them to a boil over high heat. Boil briskly for 2 minutes, remove the pan from the heat and let the beans soak for 1 hour. Now bring the water to a boil again, turn the heat down to low, and simmer the beans for 1 to 1½ hours, or until they are tender; drain and set aside. If you are using canned beans, drain them in a large sieve or colander, wash them under cold running water, then set them aside in the sieve or colander.

In a heavy skillet, heat the oil until a light haze forms over it. Add the garlic and sage and cook, stirring, for 30 seconds. Stir in the drained beans, tomatoes, salt and a few grindings of pepper. Cover and simmer over low heat for 10 minutes. Taste for seasoning, then stir in the vinegar. Serve in a heated bowl or on a deep platter.

Serves 4 to 6

Italian Broccoli Braised with White Wine (*Broccoli alla Romana*)

    ¼ cup olive oil
    1 teaspoon finely chopped garlic
    5 to 6 cups fresh broccoli flowerets (about 2 pounds fresh broccoli with stems)
    1½ cups dry white wine
    ½ teaspoon salt
    Freshly ground black pepper

In a heavy skillet, heat the olive oil until a light haze forms over it. Remove the pan from the heat and stir the garlic in the hot oil for 30 seconds. Return to moderate heat and toss the broccoli flowerets in the oil until they glisten. Add the wine, salt and a few grindings of pepper and simmer uncovered, stirring occassionally, for 5 minutes. Then cover the skillet and simmer for another 15 minutes, or until the broccoli is tender. To serve, quickly transfer the flowerets with a slotted spoon to a heated bowl or deep platter. Briskly boil the liquid left in the skillet over high heat until it has reduced to about ½ cup and pour it over the broccoli.

Serves 4 to 6

Italian Cabbage in Sweet and Sour Sauce (*Cavoli in Agrodolce*)

    3 tablespoons olive oil
    ½ cup thinly sliced onions
    1½ pounds cabbage, cut into ¼-inch strips (about 8 cups)
    3 large tomatoes, peeled, seeded and coarsely chopped
    2 tablespoons wine vinegar
    2 teaspoons salt
    Freshly ground black pepper
    1 tablespoon sugar

Heat the olive oil in a heavy skillet, add the onions and cook them over moderate heat, stirring constantly, for 2 or 3 minutes. When they are transparent but not brown, stir in the cabbage, tomatoes, vinegar, salt and a few grindings of pepper. Simmer uncovered, stirring frequently, for 20 minutes, or until the cabbage is tender. Then stir the sugar into the cabbage and cook a minute or 2 longer. Serve in a heated bowl, either preceding or along with the main course.

Serves 4 to 6

Italian Braised Peas with Prosciutto (*Piselli al Prosciutto*)

2 tablespoons butter
¼ cup finely chopped onions
2 cups fresh green peas (about 2 pounds unshelled)
¼ cup chicken stock, fresh or canned
2 ounces prosciutto, cut in 1 × ¼-inch julienne strips (about ¼ cup)
Salt
Freshly ground black pepper

In a heavy 1- to 2-quart saucepan, melt the 2 tablespoons of butter over moderate heat and cook the finely chopped onions for 7 or 8 minutes, stirring frequently until they are soft but not brown. Stir in the green peas and chicken stock, cover, and cook for 15 to 20 minutes. When the peas are tender, add the strips of prosciutto and cook, uncovered, stirring frequently, for 2 minutes more, or until all the liquid is absorbed. Taste for seasoning. Serve the peas in a heated bowl.

Note: One 10-ounce package of frozen peas may be substituted for the fresh peas. Defrost the peas thoroughly before using them, and then add them to the onions without any stock. Cook the peas uncovered, stirring frequently, for about 5 minutes, then add the prosciutto, heat through and serve.

Serves 4

Italian Braised Sweet Peppers with Tomatoes and Onions (*Peperonata*)

2 tablespoons butter
¼ cup olive oil
1 pound onions, sliced ⅛ inch thick (about 4 cups)
2 pounds green and red peppers, peeled by blanching first, seeded and cut in
    1 × ½-inch strips (about 6 cups)
2 pounds tomatoes, peeled, seeded and coarsely chopped (about 3 cups)
1 teaspoon red wine vinegar
1 teaspoon salt
Freshly ground black pepper

In a heavy skillet, melt the 2 tablespoons of butter with the ¼ cup of olive oil over moderate heat. Add the onions and cook them, turning them frequently, for 10 minutes, or until they are soft and lightly browned. Stir in the peppers, reduce the heat, cover the skillet and cook for 10 minutes. Add the tomatoes, vinegar, salt and a few grindings of black pepper; cover and cook for another 5 minutes.

Then cook the vegetables uncovered over high heat, stirring gently, until almost all the liquid has boiled away.

Serve, as a hot vegetable dish, preceding or along with the main course.

Serves 6

Indian Style Vegetable Curries

Indian style vegetable curries compose the original Indian recipes. These may be too spicy for many Westerners and even some Easterners. Adjustments of the amount of spices are recommended according to individual taste, unless one enjoys very hot spicy food. Generally, be cautious with spices the first time you try a recipe, and increase the spices according to your taste in later preparations of the same or similar dishes. Vegetable curries are normally eaten with rice, or home-made Indian bread—*chapati* or *puri*. The recipes for cooking rice including gourmet pilaus/pilaf, as well as for chapati and puri are given in the next section on 'grains.' Arabian or pitta bread can go very well (after heating in the oven) with most of these vegetable curries and provide a convenient substitute for chapati or puri. Yogurt dishes, chutney and salad are often served with the main meal.

An appropriate combination of Indian vegetarian foods may contain:
Rice pilau (pilaf) or wholewheat bread such as chapati, puri, parautha
Vegetable curry
One of the beans such as black beans, chickpeas or soup such as hot lentil soup (sambar)
Salad
Yogurt dish (Rayta)
Chutney
Sweet Dessert (such as gajar halva, or khir)

Fresh Ginger, Bell Pepper and Tomato Curry (*Adarak Simla-Mirch Tamatar Tarkari*)

8 ounces bell pepper
2 ounces sliced fresh ginger root
½ teaspoonful white pepper
1 pound tomatoes
Chopped fresh coriander leaves
2 teaspoonfuls sugar
2 teaspoonfuls salt
½ cup cooking oil

Heat the cooking oil. Add finely-sliced bell pepper, 1 teaspoonful salt and ¼ teaspoonful white pepper and stir for a few minutes or until the bell pepper is half-cooked. Add wedges of the tomatoes, sliced ginger, the remaining salt, white pepper and two teaspoonfuls sugar. Cook, stirring occasionally and carefully, so that the pieces of tomato remain firm and do not turn into a purée.

Serve immediately, sprinkled with chopped coriander leaves or parsley.

Eggplant and Bell Pepper Curry (*Baingan Simla-Mirch Tarkari*)

2 ounces cooking oil
12 ounces eggplant
4 ounces onions
2 teaspoonfuls salt
½ teaspoonful allspice (*garam masala*)
12 ounces bell pepper
½ teaspoonful red pepper
Chopped fresh coriander leaves

Heat the cooking oil. Add roughly-cut onions and cook for a few minutes. Then add sliced eggplant and bell pepper. Stir for a few minutes; add salt and the red pepper and cook on low heat until three-quarters cooked. Lastly add slices of skinned tomatoes and cook till tender.

Serve sprinkled with allspice and chopped coriander leaves or parsley.

Green Peas and Mushrooms (*Khumbi and Mattar Bhaji*)

1 pound fresh mushrooms
3 tablespoons clarified butter or cooking oil
½ teaspoon black mustard seeds
1½ cups finely chopped onions
1 teaspoon allspice (*garam masala*)
½ teaspoon turmeric
½ cup unflavored yogurt
1 cup fresh green peas or 1 ten-ounce package frozen green peas, thoroughly defrosted and drained
1 teaspoon salt
3 tablespoons finely chopped fresh coriander

Wipe the mushrooms with a damp paper towel and cut away the tough ends of the stems. With a small, sharp knife, cut the mushrooms lengthwise into paper-thin slices. Set aside.

In a heavy skillet or a 12-inch wok, heat 3 tablespoons of the cooking oil over moderate heat. Add the mustard seeds and stir for 15 seconds to coat the seeds with oil, then add the onions and, stirring almost constantly, fry for 7 to 8 minutes, or until the onions are soft and golden brown. Watch carefully for any sign of burning and regulate heat accordingly.

Stir in the allspice and turmeric, then add the yogurt and bring to a boil. Add the peas and salt and, stirring constantly, cook for 3 minutes. Then add the mushrooms and 1 tablespoon of the coriander. Reduce the heat to the lowest possible point, cover tightly, and simmer for 15 minutes, or until the peas and mushrooms are tender. Taste for seasoning.

To serve, transfer the entire contents of the pan to a heated bowl or platter

and sprinkle the top with the remaining 2 tablespoons of coriander.
Serves 4

Tomato and Eggplant Curry (dry) (*Tamatar Baingan*)

    1 pound eggplant
    2 ounces cooking oil
    12 ounces tomato
    $\frac{1}{2}$ teaspoonful white pepper
    $\frac{1}{2}$ teaspoonful red pepper
    3 to 4 ounces thinly-sliced onions
    $2\frac{1}{2}$ teaspoonfuls salt
    2 to 3 shredded green peppers (optional)

Peel and cut the eggplant into wedges. Rub on $1\frac{1}{2}$ teaspoonfuls salt and leave them in a colander for half an hour to allow the moisture to drip. Wipe each piece carefully but do not wash.

Heat the cooking oil; sprinkle $\frac{1}{2}$ teaspoonful red pepper, stir for a second and add sliced onions. Cook on low heat so that it does not brown. Then add the eggplant; cover and cook on low heat until they are half done. Lastly add slices of peeled seeded tomatoes, green peppers, the remaining salt and the white pepper. Cover and cook on low heat until done. Shake the pan every now and then whilst cooking in order to avoid sticking of the eggplant or the spices to the bottom of the pan.

Potato, Tomato and Onion Curry (*Alu Tamatar Piaz Tarkari*)

    1 pound small potatoes (marble-sized)
    1 pound tomatoes
    2 teaspoonfuls salt
    $\frac{1}{2}$ teaspoonful red pepper
    $\frac{1}{2}$ teaspoonful turmeric
    4 to 6 tablespoons cooking oil
    8 ounces small-sized whole onions
    $\frac{1}{2}$ teaspoonful (*garam masala*) allspice
    1 ounce finely-cut ginger root
    1 teaspoonful sugar

Heat the cooking oil. Skin the onions and, keeping them whole, cook on medium heat for half an hour. Add small-sized whole potatoes or roughly-cut large ones, salt, red pepper and turmeric and cook on low heat. Do not add any liquid but cover the pan with a saucer-shaped lid and keep some water on it. When the potatoes are nearly cooked, add wedges of the tomatoes, sliced green pepper and ginger and the sugar. Raise the heat from medium to high and continue cooking. The potatoes and tomatoes, though cooked, should remain firm.

Serve sprinkled with allspice (*garam masala*) and chopped fresh coriander leaves or parsley.

Spinach and Broccoli Purée (*Sag*)

> 1 cup water
> ½ pound fresh spinach, washed trimmed and coarsely chopped
> ½ pound fresh broccoli including the stalks, washed, trimmed and coarsely chopped
> 3 tablespoons clarified butter or cooking oil
> 1 tablespoon scraped, finely chopped fresh ginger root
> ½ cup finely chopped onions
> 1 teaspoon salt
> ¼ teaspoon ground cumin
> ¼ teaspoon turmeric
> ½ teaspoon ground coriander
> ½ teaspoon allspice *(garam masala)*

Combine ½ cup of the water and a handful of the spinach in the jar of an electric blender, and blend at high speed for 30 seconds, or until the mixture is reduced to a smooth purée. Turn the machine off and scrape down the sides of the jar with a rubber spatula. Then add another handful of spinach, purée for 30 seconds, and stop the machine again. Repeat until all the spinach has been puréed. Transfer the spinach to a bowl, and pour the remaining ½ cup of water into the blender jar. Purée the broccoli a handful at a time as you did the spinach, then stir the puréed broccoli into the spinach.

In a heavy skillet or wok, heat the cooking oil or clarified butter over moderate heat. Add the ginger and fry for 1 minute. Add the onions and salt and continue to fry, lifting and turning the mixture constantly, for 7 to 8 minutes or until the onions are soft and golden brown.

Stirring after each addition, add the cumin, turmeric, coriander and allspice (*garam masala*). Fry for 1 or 2 minutes, until the ingredients are well combined, then stir in the spinach and broccoli a cup or so at a time and fry for 5 minutes more. Reduce the heat to the lowest possible point and stirring, occasionally, simmer uncovered for 15 minutes, until almost all of the liquid has evaporated and the mixture leaves the sides of the pan in a solid mass. Serve at once from a heated bowl or platter.

In the Punjab, where it originated, *sag* is usually made with fresh mustard greens; you may substitute these for the spinach and broccoli or broccoli alone.

Serves 4 to 6

Fresh Green Beans with Coconut (*Same ki Bhaji*)

> 4 tablespoons clarified butter or cooking oil
> 1 teaspoon black mustard seeds
> 2 tablespoons split black beans (*urad dal,* if available)
> ½ cup finely chopped onions
> 1 teaspoon scraped, finely chopped fresh ginger root
> 1 teaspoon salt
> ½ teaspoon freshly ground black pepper
> 1 pound fresh green string beans, trimmed and cut crosswise into paper-thin rounds

¼ teaspoon ground red pepper
¼ cup finely grated fresh coconut (if available)
2 tablespoons finely chopped fresh coriander
2 tablespoons fresh lemon juice

In a heavy skillet, or wok, heat the clarified butter or cooking oil over moderate heat. Add the mustard seeds and fry *urad dal* for 3 minutes, until the dal browns lightly. (If dal is not available, fry the mustard seeds alone for 30 seconds.) Thoroughly stir in the onions, ginger, salt and pepper, and drop in the green beans. Stirring constantly, add the red pepper and fry 5 minutes longer. Add the coconut and coriander, reduce the heat to low, and cover the pan. Stirring occasionally, cook for 10 minutes more, or until the beans are tender. Sprinkle with lemon juice, taste for seasoning, and serve at once.
　　Serves 4

Fried Potato Curry (*Dam Alu*)

1½ pound potatoes
4 ounces grated onions
10 cloves of garlic
½ teaspoonful turmeric
1 teaspoonful white cumin seeds
1 tablespoonful coriander seeds
12 peppercorns
½ ounce almonds
2 teaspoonfuls salt
1 cup yogurt
½ teaspoonful allspice *(garam masala)*
2 cups of cooking oil for frying the potatoes
1 teaspoonful red pepper
1 teaspoonful poppy seeds
6 cloves
2 brown cardamoms
½ ounce shredded coconut
5 green cardamoms or a little mace
¼ cup water
1 tablespoonful chopped fresh coriander leaves or parsley
2 finely-cut green pepper

Select potatoes of the size of walnuts. Peel and prick all over with a fork and soak in 2½ cups of water and 2 teaspoonfuls salt for about half an hour. Dry the potatoes in a clean dry cloth. Heat 2 cups cooking oil and fry the potatoes on medium heat till browned on all sides. While the potatoes are frying, roast coriander seeds on a hot griddle, and sift the skins. Also roast poppy seeds, coconut, almonds, cumin seeds, cloves, peppercorns, brown cardamoms and the mace or nutmeg. Grind these along with the ginger, garlic and a little water till they are converted into a fine paste.

Heat ½ cup cooking oil and brown the grated onions. Remove the pan from the heat, add red pepper, turmeric, crushed green cardamoms, salt and the ground paste to the browned onions. Then cook on low heat. Beat 1 cup yogurt lightly and add a little of it at a time to the mixture until about half is used up. Add fried potatoes and cook for another five minutes. Then add the remaining yogurt and ½ cup hot water. Keep it in the oven or cook on low heat for about 20 minutes.

This is a potato preparation of distinction in which whole potatoes are cooked in spices. The spices which adhere to the potatoes not only give them a very good taste but also make them exceedingly presentable in appearance.

Homemade Cheese with Peas (*Mattar Panir*)

Cheese

2 quarts milk
½ cup unflavored yogurt
2 tablespoons fresh strained lemon juice

Peas

5 tablespoons clarified butter or cooking oil
2 tablespoons scraped, finely chopped fresh ginger root
1 tablespoon finely chopped garlic
1 cup finely chopped onions
1 teaspoon salt
1 teaspoon turmeric
¼ teaspoon ground hot red pepper
1 teaspoon ground coriander
1 tablespoon allspice *(garam masala)*
2 cups finely chopped fresh tomatoes
1½ cups fresh green peas or 1 ten-ounce package frozen peas, thoroughly defrosted
1 teaspoon sugar (optional)
3 tablespoons finely chopped fresh coriander

Prepare the cheese in the following fashion: In a heavy 3- to 4-quart saucepan, bring the milk to a boil over high heat. As soon as the foam begins to rise, remove the pan from the heat and gently but thoroughly stir in the yogurt and lemon juice. The curds will begin to solidify immediately and separate from the liquid whey.

Pour the entire contents of the pan into a large sieve set over a bowl and lined with a double thickness of cheese-cloth. Let the curds drain undisturbed until the cloth is cool enough to handle. Then wrap the cloth tightly around the curds and wring it vigorously to squeeze out all the excess liquid. Reserve 1 cup of the whey in the bowl and discard the rest.

Place the cheese, still wrapped in cheesecloth, on a cutting board and set another board or large flat-bottomed skillet on top of it. Weight the top with canned foods, heavy pots or the like, weighing in all about 15 pounds, and let it rest in this fashion at room temperature for 6 to 8 hours, or until the cheese is firm and compact. Unwrap the cheese, cut it into ½ inch cubes, cover with wax paper or plastic wrap, and refrigerate until ready to use. (There should be about 1 to 1½ cups of cheese cubes.)

To prepare the cheese and peas, heat the cooking oil in a heavy skillet. Add the cheese cubes and fry them for 4 or 5 minutes, turning the cubes about gently but constantly with a slotted spoon until they are golden brown on all sides. As they brown, transfer the cubes of cheese to a plate.

Add the ginger and garlic to the cooking oil remaining in the skillet and, stirring constantly, fry for 30 seconds. Add the onions and salt and, stirring occasionally, continue to fry for 7 or 8 minutes, or until the onions are soft and golden brown. Watch carefully for any signs of burning and regulate the heat accordingly.

Stir in ¼ cup of the reserved whey, then add the turmeric, red pepper, ground coriander and allspice (*garam masala*). When they are well blended, stir in the remaining ¼ cup of whey and the tomatoes, and bring to a boil over high heat. Reduce the heat to low and simmer partially covered for 10 minutes, stirring occasionally. Add the peas and taste for seasoning. If the gravy has too acid a flavor add up to 1 teaspoon sugar.

Remove the cover, stirring occasionally, cook for 3 minutes. Then add the cheese cubes and 1 tablespoon of the fresh coriander, cover the skillet tightly, and simmer over low heat for 10 to 20 minutes, or longer if you are using fresh peas and they are not yet tender.

To serve, transfer the entire contents of the pan to a heated bowl or deep platter and garnish the top with the remaining 2 tablespoons of chopped fresh coriander.

Serves 4 to 6

Bean Recipes

The first six recipes given here are Indian style gourmet cooking. You notice high use of cooking oil or preferably clarified butter (*ghee*). For weight watchers these recipes can be modified by eliminating or reducing use of fat as given for lentils in the last recipe. Legumes are not a complete protein alone as discussed in Chapter 5 and needs to be combined with a whole grain. These are usually served with chapati (see Indian bread recipes) or rice.

Whole Black Beans (*Urhad* or *Maanh Sabat*)

  8 ounces whole black beans
  2½ to 3 teaspoonfuls salt
  1 ounce finely-cut ginger root
  4 dried red pepper
  4 cups of water

12 finely-cut cloves of garlic
½ ounce clarified butter or cooking oil

Ingredients for frying in cooking oil:

2 ounces clarified butter or cooking oil
3 finely-cut green pepper (seeds removed)
½ teaspoon allspice *(garam masala)*
1 ounce finely-cut ginger
½ teaspoonful red pepper

For cooking the beans: Remove the grit from the beans and wash them 3 to 4 times. Boil the water and add salt, beans, garlic, ginger, red pepper and cooking oil. Cover with a saucer-shaped lid containing a little water. When it comes to a boil, reduce the heat and simmer for 3 to 4 hours. Alternatively pressure-cook at 15 pounds pressure for half an hour; and allow the pressure to drop by itself; uncover, cook the beans further in the same pan or another open pan on low heat for half an hour; stir and mash them every now and then till they are reduced to a creamy consistency.

For frying (*tadka or baghar*): Heat the clarified butter or cooking oil, add ginger, stir for a second and then add green pepper, red pepper and the allspice. (*garam masala*) Mix half of it into the cooked black beans (*urhad*) and keep the remaining half for adding to it just before serving.

Black beans (*urhad*) is a North Indian dish and is taken with chapaties (see Indian breads) or plain boiled rice.

Whole Green Beans or Mung Beans (*Moong Sabat*)

Ingredients for cooking the beans:

8 ounces whole green beans
2½ to 3 teaspoonfuls salt
1 ounce finely-cut ginger root
4 dried red pepper
4 cups water
12 finely-cut cloves of garlic
½ ounce clarified butter or cooking oil
1 teaspoonful turmeric

Ingredients for frying (*baghar* or *tadka*):
The same as described above for black beans except for the addition of 2 ounces finely-cut onions.

For cooking: The procedure is the same as described above for whole black beans.
For frying (*baghar* or *tadka*): Heat the clarified butter or cooking oil, fry the

onions till golden brown and add ginger and the green pepper. Stir and add red pepper and the allspice (*garam masala*). Mix half of it into the cooked beans and keep the remaining half for addition to it just before serving.

Chick-peas (*Kabli Channas*)

> **8 ounces chick-peas** (*kabli channas*)
> **1½ teaspoonfuls of salt**
> **3 ounces cooking oil**
> **½ ounce ginger**
> **4 cloves**
> **2½ ounces grated onions**
> **4 ounces tomatoes**
> **1 or 2 green pepper**
> **½ teaspoonful allspice** (*garam masala*)
> **3 cups water**
> **12 cloves of garlic**
> **½ teaspoonful white cumin seeds**
> **2 brown cardamoms (seeds only)**
> **1 inch (2½ centimeter) piece of cinnamon** (*darchini*)
> **½ teaspoonful red pepper**
> **1 teaspoonful dry coriander seeds**
> **1 tablespoonful chopped coriander leaves**

Pick, wash and soak the chick-peas overnight in 3 cups of water. Add 1 teaspoonful of salt and 1 or 2 green pepper and simmer till tender. Alternatively pressure-cook at 15 pounds pressure for 10 minutes and allow the pressure to drop by itself.

Heat the cooking oil and fry the shredded onions. Remove from the heat when golden brown, add ½ teaspoonful red pepper, stir and keep it on the heat again. Continue frying the onions, adding a little water at a time till 2 tablespoonfuls are consumed. Then add the remaining spices, ginger and the garlic ground together. Fry for 5 minutes or till the cooking oil separates from the spices. Add the roughly-cut tomatoes and stir till they form a homogenous mixture with the spices. Then add the boiled chick-peas and fry on low heat for 10 minutes whilst adding the chick-peas stock, a little at a time. After adding the last of the stock, simmer on low heat for 20 minutes.

Serve, sprinkled with allspice (*garam masala*) and chopped fresh coriander leaves or parsley.

Chick-peas (sour) (*Khatta Kabali Channas*)

Ingredients for soaking:

> **8 ounces chickpeas**
> **2 cups water**
> **½ teaspoonful bicarbonate soda**

Ingredients for boiling:

> 8 ounces soaked chick-peas and the water in which they are soaked
> 1 chopped green pepper
> 4 cloves of garlic
> 12 peppercorns
> 6 cloves
> 2 ounces onions
> ½ ounce chopped ginger
> 4 cardamoms
> 1 inch piece cinnamon stick
> 1 teaspoonful salt

Ingredients for sour chick-peas:

> 4 ounces clarified butter or cooking oil
> 8 cloves of garlic
> Chick-peas stock (water separated from chick-peas)
> ½ to ¾ powdered dried green mango
> 1½ ounces sliced ginger
> 4 ounces sliced onions
> 1 teaspoonful red pepper
> Cooked chick-peas
> ½ to ¾ ounce dried pomegranate seeds
> 3 to 4 sliced green pepper
> ½ teaspoonful salt

Ingredients for sprinkling over:

> 1 teaspoonful ground roasted black cumin seeds
> 1 to 2 ounces sizzling hot cooking oil
> 1 teaspoonful allspice *(garam masala)*
> 1 tablespoonful finely-chopped coriander seeds

Ingredients for garnishing:

> Wedges of tomatoes
> A few onion rings
> Cooked small potatoes
> A few green pepper

Wash and soak the chick-peas overnight in 2 cups water containing ½ teaspoonful bicarbonate of soda (baking soda). Boil them in the same water and add 1 teaspoonful salt, 2 ounces finely-chopped onions, 1 chopped green pepper, ½ ounce chopped ginger, 4 cloves of garlic, 4 cardamoms, 2 peppercorns, 1 inch (2½ centimeter) piece of cinnamon and 6 cloves. Simmer in a pan for about 1 hour or until tender. An alternative is to pressure-cook for 7 minutes at 15 pounds pressure. Reduce pressure immediately by putting wet duster over the lid. The chick-peas should remain whole after they are cooked. Separate the chickpeas from the stock and discard whole spices, ginger, garlic and onions.

Heat 4 ounces clarified butter or cooking oil. Add 4 ounces thinly-sliced onions and 8 thinly-sliced cloves of garlic. Brown. Remove from the heat, add 1 teaspoonful red pepper and then ⅓ of the stock of the chick-peas. Cook till the mixture browns, the stock dries up and the onions become a thick purée. Add the chick-peas and 3 ounces of the chick-peas stock, stir and simmer on low heat for 10 minutes, stirring very carefully, so that they do not break. Mix powdered dried green mango, ground roasted pomegranate seeds, 1½ ounces sliced ginger, 3 slices green pepper and salt. Leave on very low heat for about 15 to 20 minutes so that the flavor of the spices penetrates the chick-peas. Pour 1 or 2 ounces sizzling clarified butter over the chick-peas.

Serve hot, sprinkled with roasted powdered black cumin seeds, allspice (*garam masala*) and chopped coriander leaves. Garnish with wedges of tomatoes, cooked potato bits, a few onion rings and whole green pepper.

Curried Red Kidney Beans (*Rajma Dal*)

> 2 cups dried red kidney beans *(rajma dal)*
> 3 quarts water
> 1 tablespoon turmeric
> ¼ teaspoon ground hot red pepper
> 1 tablespoon salt
> ¼ cup vegetable oil
> 1 cup finely chopped onions
> 3 tablespoons scraped, finely chopped fresh ginger root
> 1 tablespoon finely chopped garlic
> 2 tablespoons ground coriander
> 1 teaspoon ground cumin
> 1 teaspoon allspice *(garam masala)*
> 3 medium-sized firm ripe tomatoes, washed and coarsely chopped
> 4 tablespoons finely chopped fresh coriander
> 3 tablespoons clarified butter or cooking oil

In a large sieve or colander, wash the kidney beans under cold running water until the draining water runs clear. Drop the beans into a heavy 4- to 5-quart saucepan, pour in enough water to cover them by 1 inch, and bring to a boil over high heat. Boil briskly for 2 minutes, then remove the pan from the heat and let the beans soak uncovered for 1 hour.

Drain the beans in a colander and add 3 quarts of fresh cold water to the saucepan. Add the beans, then stir in the turmeric, red pepper and salt, and bring to a boil over high heat. Reduce the heat to low, partially cover the pan, and simmer for 3 hours, or until the beans are tender but still intact. Drain the beans in a sieve or colander set over a deep bowl and set the beans and cooking liquid aside.

In a heavy 5- to 6-quart casserole, heat the vegetable oil over high heat until a light haze forms above it. Drop in the onions, ginger and garlic, and lower the heat to moderate. Stirring constantly, fry the mixture for 7 or 8 minutes, or until the onions are soft and golden brown. Watch carefully for any sign of burning and regulate the heat accordingly.

Add the ground coriander, cumin and allspice (*garam masala*), and fry for 30 seconds, stirring constantly. Still stirring, add the tomatoes and cook over moderate heat for 5 minutes, until most of the liquid in the pan evaporates and the mixture is thick enough to draw away from the sides and bottom of the pan in a dense mass. Pour in the bean cooking liquid, add 2 tablespoons of the fresh coriander and bring to a boil, stirring occasionally. Cover tightly and simmer for 10 minutes.

Stir in the beans and cook for a few minutes to heat them through. Taste for seasoning, ladle the entire contents of the pan into a heated bowl or tureen, and sprinkle the top with the clarified butter (optional) and the remaining 2 tablespoons of fresh coriander. Serve at once.

Serves 6 to 8

Indian Hot Lentil and Vegetable Soup (*Sambar*)

Ingredients for cooking the lentil and the vegetables:

> ½ cup lentil or split peas or dried pigeon peas *(arhar dal)*
> 1 carrot
> 1 teaspoonful turmeric
> 1½ cups water
> 1 potato
> 1 eggplant
> 1½ teaspoonfuls salt
> 1 teaspoonful cooking oil

Ingredients to be added after the soup is cooked:

> 1 ounce tamarind pulp (get from Oriental store, if available)
> 1 teaspoonful coriander seeds
> ¼ coconut
> A grain of asafoetida of the size of a peppercorn (if available)
> ½ teaspoonful white cumin seeds

Ingredients for seasoning the soup:

> 2 to 4 tablespoons cooking oil
> A few bits of red pepper
> 8 to 10 small curry leaves
> ½ teaspoonful red hot pepper
> 1 teaspoonful mustard seeds
> 2 finely-cut green pepper
> 1 teaspoonful curry powder

Wash and soak lentil or split peas for half an hour. Drain. Boil in 1½ cup water with carrot, potato, salt and turmeric till the split peas become tender. Discard the carrot and the potato. Dice the eggplant and put it back into the pan. If other vegetables like marrow or okra are used in place of the eggplant dice them also. Squeeze the tamarind pulp and add to the boiled soup. Simmer for 10 minutes. Heat the cooking oil and fry cumin seeds, coriander seeds, asafoetida and the coconut. Remove these from the cooking oil and grind into a fine paste. In the remaining, fry mustard seeds, finely-cut green pepper and curry leaves or two bay leaves and bits of red pepper. Add the ground paste and cook for 5 minutes. Before serving, season the soup prepared above with the fried ingredients and *sambar* powder. If it is thick add a little boiling water and salt if required and reheat all to boiling point.

Serve hot with boiled rice or wholewheat bread.

Basic Lentils

> **1 cup lentils, washed**
> **2 cups water**
> **³⁄₄ teaspoon salt**
> **2 bay leaves**
> **¼ cup chopped onion**
> **¼ cup chopped green pepper**
> **¼ cup chopped or sliced celery**
> **1 clove of garlic minced**
> **½ teaspoon cumin, ground**

Combine all ingredients in pot and cook, covered, over medium heat for about 30 minutes or until lentils are tender.

Lentils, like most other legumes are not a complete protein alone and needs to be combined with a whole grain. Lentils are usually served with chapati or rice.

This recipe is suggested to slow down aging.

GRAINS

Cracked Wheat Cereal*

> **½ cup cracked wheat**
> **2 cups water**

Bring the water to a rolling boil; stir in the cracked wheat. Lower the heat so that mixture cooks slowly. Cook approximately 20 to 25 minutes, stirring from time to time, until mixture thickens sufficiently. (Cover near end of cooking time if a softer texture is desired.)

Serve plain, or with a light sprinkling of cinnamon, and/or sliced fruit, if desired.
Serves 1 or 2

Sesame Crackers

> **1½ cups wholewheat flour**
> **¼ cup soy flour**

¼ **cup sesame seeds**
¾ **teaspoon salt**
⅓ **cup oil**
½ **cup water (as needed)**

Stir the flours, seeds, and salt together. Add the oil and blend well. Add enough water so that the dough can be kneaded into a soft ball and can be rolled easily to a thickness of ⅛ inch . Cut the dough into cracker shapes and place on an ungreased sheet. Bake at 350° F. (180° C.) for about 15 to 20 minutes or until the crackers are crisp and golden.

Makes 3 to 4 dozen crackers

Oatmeal*

1 cup "old fashioned" rolled oats
2 cups water

Bring 2 cups of water to a rolling boil; stir in the oats. Lower the heat so that the mixture cooks slowly. Cook approximately 12 to 15 minutes, stirring from time to time, until the mixture thickens sufficiently. (Cover near the end of cooking time if a softer texture is desired.)

Serve plain, or with a light sprinkling of cinnamon, if desired, and/or sliced fruit.

Serves 1 or 2

Oatmeal with Stewed Apples

2 cups "old fashioned" rolled oats
2 cups boiling water
1 apple, thinly sliced
¼ **teaspoon ground cinnamon**
Skim milk

Stir the oats into boiling water in the top of a double boiler; cook and stir for several minutes. Add the apples and the cinnamon. Cook 10 minutes, mixing occasionally. Serve hot with skim milk.

Serves 4

RICE PILAUS (PIRAF)

Basic Curried Lentils with Rice

3 large onions, chopped
½ **cup vegetable oil**
1 cup lentils
1 cup brown rice
6 to 7 cups water

1 tablespoon salt
1½ teaspoons curry powder
Minced parsley, to garnish

Cook onions in oil until soft and golden, and set aside. Meanwhile cook lentils and rice in water for 35 minutes. Add salt, curry powder, and onions. Cook another 20 minutes or until most of water is absorbed. Garnish with minced parsley.

Basic Pilau Rice

1 medium onion, chopped
½ cup raisins
1 tablespoon pine nuts
1½ cups raw rice
1 cup yogurt
5 tablespoons butter
¼ teaspoon chili powder
2 teaspoon salt
¼ teaspoon powdered cardamom
½ teaspoon powdered ginger
2 teaspoons mustard seeds
3¼ cups water
1 clove garlic, minced

In pot, sauté onion, garlic, raisins, nuts, salt, and spices in butter for 5 minutes.
   Add rice, and continue to sauté, over low heat, stirring, for 7 minutes.
   Add yogurt. Pour in water. Cover. Cook over low heat until rice is done (about 15 minutes).

Basic Rice and Fried Beans

1 cup raw garbanzo beans
3 cups onions, chopped
2 cloves garlic, minced
2 tablespoons vegetable oil
1½ cups wine
2 teaspoons ginger
2 cups raw rice, cooked according to directions

Cook beans. Heat chopped onions in oven for a few minutes at 300° F. (150° C.). Sauté onions and garlic in oil and small amount of wine until slightly brown. Add beans while still hot. Add ginger and remainder of wine, and simmer until beans are slightly brown. Pour over rice and serve. Kidney beans, pintos, and black beans are also tasty when fried.
   Makes 6 servings

Black Beans on Rice

1 pound dry black beans

6 cups boiling water
2 green peppers, chopped
6–8 green onions (scallions) with tops, chopped
1 clove garlic, minced
⅓ cup oil
2 teaspoons salt; seasonings (optional)
1 pound brown rice, cooked

Cover the beans with the boiling water and cook for 1 hour. Sauté the green peppers, green onions (reserve for 1 to 2 tablespoons), and garlic in oil. Combine the vegetables with the beans, add the salt and other seasonings (as desired), and cook until the beans are tender and the liquid is thick. Serve over brown rice. Garnish with the reserved chopped green onions.

Serves 16, ¾ cup each

Soy and Brown-Rice Loaf

2 cups cooked mashed soybeans
1 cup cooked brown rice
1 cup milk
½ cup enriched bread crumbs
1 tablespoon oil
1 tablespoon powdered vegetable broth
2 tablespoons minced onion
Salt, as desired (optional)

Mix all the ingredients well. Place in an oiled loaf pan. Bake in a 350° F. (180° C.) oven for 45 minutes. If desired, moisten the top of the loaf with tomato sauce.

Serves 4

Rice and Mushroom Ring

1 cup raw wild rice
4 cups water
1 pound fresh mushrooms, sliced
½ cup dry white wine
⅛ teaspoon ground nutmeg
⅛ teaspoon ground pepper

Wash the raw rice thoroughly. Bring water to a boil; add rice, reduce heat to low, and cover saucepan. Simmer the rice for 40 minutes, fluffing it occasionally with a fork. Meanwhile, simmer the mushrooms in a skillet with the white wine, nutmeg, and pepper, until the wine has almost evaporated. Combine the cooked rice and the mushrooms. Pack the rice mixture into a 1-quart nonstick ring mold. Set the mold into a pan of water and place it on the middle rack of the oven. Bake at 350° F. (180° C.) for 30 minutes. Unmold the ring on a large round platter. Fill the center with steamed green peas, if desired.

Serves 4 to 6

INDIAN STYLE RICE PILAUS

Cauliflower Pilau (*Gobi Pilau*)

>   9 ounces rice
>   3 ounces clarified butter or cooking oil
>   2 teaspoonfuls salt
>   2 ounces onions
>   12 finely-chopped cloves of garlic
>   2 crushed brown cardamoms
>   1 inch piece of cinnamon stick
> $3/4$ teaspoonful allspice *(garam masala)*
>   2 cups hot water
>   8 ounces cauliflower sprigs
>   5 tablespoonfuls sour cream
> $1/2$ ounce ginger
>   2 to 3 green pepper
>   6 cloves
>   1 teaspoonful black cumin seeds *(kala zeera)*
> $1/2$ teaspoonful red pepper

Ingredients for garnishing:

>   2 ounces thinly-sliced fried onions
>   Finely-chopped fresh coriander leaves or parsley
>   4 ounces fried potato vermicelli (optional)
>   Sliced tomatoes and cucumber
> $1/2$ ounce roasted almonds

Clean and wash the rice. Soak for half an hour in 2 cups water. Heat the cooking oil, fry the garnished (except the tomatoes and cucumber) and keep them aside. Fry the cauliflower sprigs with a little salt and pepper sprinkled over them, till they are half-cooked. Remove them from the cooking oil and fry the onions and garlic. Add brown cardamoms, cinnamon, cloves and the rice, fry for a few minutes more and then add the fried sprigs, sliced ginger, green pepper, red pepper, salt, black cumin seeds and *garam masala*. Continue frying the mixture for about 5 minutes, add water in which the rice was previously soaked and lastly add the cream. Cover and cook in a pressure cooker or in a pan.

Garnish and serve with yogurt or a curry.

Rice-Peas Pilau (*Mattar Pilau*)

>   9 ounces rice
>   3 ounces clarified butter or cooking oil
> $1/2$ ounce ginger root
> $1\frac{1}{2}$ teaspoonfuls salt
>   6 cloves
>   12 peppercorns (optional)

2 to 3 green pepper
1 teaspoonful allspice *(garam masala)*
2 cups hot water
6 ounces peas
2 ounces finely-sliced onions
12 finely-chopped cloves of garlic
2 brown cardamom pods
1 inch piece of cinnamon
1 teaspoonful black cumin seeds
½ teaspoonful red pepper

Ingredients for garnishing:

2 teaspoonfuls chopped fresh coriander leaves or parsley
Slices of the hard-boiled egg (optional)
2 ounces thinly-sliced fried onions
Sliced tomatoes and cucumber
½ ounce roasted almonds

Clean, wash and soak the rice for half an hour in 2 cups water. Heat the *ghee* (cooking oil) and fry without stirring 2 ounces thinly-sliced onions. Shake the frying pan to prevent the onions from burning. When crisp and golden brown remove from the cooking oil. Fry the almonds till they are crisp but not burnt. Keep both the onions and the almonds in a warm place for subsequent garnishing.

Heat the cooking oil, fry 2 ounces finely-sliced onions and the garlic. When the onions are golden brown in color add cardamoms, cinnamon, cloves and pepper-corns and stir for 2 to 3 minutes. (These are added whole and are not removed before the pilau is served. They are, however, not eaten.) Add peas and continue frying for 5 minutes. Then add rice, salt, red pepper, black cumin seeds and the *garam masala* and fry the mixture for another 5 minutes. Add water in which the rice was previously soaked, the thinly-sliced ginger, and green pepper. Cook over medium heat till half the water in the rice dries up. Then reduce the heat to low; cover the top of the pan with a double-folded cloth, place the lid over that and cook on low heat till the grains become soft. Remove the cloth, and leave in the oven at warm till the rice is served.

Serve in oval dish. Cover the center of rice with fried onions and almonds and arrange alternate slices of cucumber, eggs and tomatoes on the sides. Sprinkle chopped coriander leaves or parsley all over. Whipped yogurt or vegetable curry can be served with it.

Vegetable Fried Rice (*Sabzi Pilau*)

This is the vegetarian counterpart of the Chinese young chow fried rice. Black mushrooms are used in place of pork, white mushrooms instead of prawns and the Indian cream cheese (*panir*) replaces the eggs. Other ingredients are the same as those used in preparation of young chow fried rice and the method of cooking is also similar.

Ingredients:

9 ounces rice (boiled in 2 cups water)
1 ounce white mushrooms
½ ounce black mushrooms
4 ounces Indian cream cheese *(panir)*
4 ounces carrots
4 ounces peas
Green stalks of 2 spring onions
2 finely chopped green pepper
2 teaspoonfuls salt
½ teaspoonful white pepper
4 ounces cooking oil

Wash, soak and boil the rice, preferably a day or at least a few hours before it is required, and keep it in a colander overnight. This dries the rice and causes the grains to separate from each other. If, however, the rice is to be cooked within a few hours, fry in 2 teaspoonfuls melted butter for 3 to 4 minutes as this preliminary frying keeps the rice grains separate. Then add the necessary quantity of water and cook over medium heat. Cool the rice by keeping it in a colander.

Soak the white mushrooms in hot water for about 3 to 4 hours and then clean them very thoroughly under running water. Boil them for about half an hour or till they are tender. Pour boiling hot water over the black mushrooms and boil for 2 minutes. Chop both types of mushrooms separately.

Set the *panir* by keeping it under some weight, chop it very fine and give it a yellowish tinge similar to that of an egg yolk by the addition of a bit of yellow coloring. Chop the spring onions. Boil the whole carrots till half-cooked and dice them into cubes of the size of peas. Chop the pepper finely.

Heat 2 teaspoonfuls cooking oil and a pinch of salt. Add white mushrooms and fry on a high heat for 5 minutes. Take them out, add a little more cooking oil and the salt and fry the black mushrooms. Similarly fry the Indian cream cheese (*panir*), peas, carrots, spring onions and green pepper separately. Wash and dry the pan every time. Heat the remaining cooking oil and 1 teaspoonful salt and lightly fry the rice. Then add all the fried ingredients and ½ teaspoonful white pepper. Continue stirring for 10 minutes. Add a little more salt if necessary. Mix thoroughly.

Serve in a hot China dish immediately after preparation. Do not cover as condensed steam makes the rice soggy. Provide chilli sauce separately. Before serving sprinkle on ½ teaspoonful black pepper.

Properly cooked fried rice is always dry and is not messy. It is essential that the preparation of the fried rice should be completed only a few minutes before serving. If brown rice is preferred, mix two teaspoonfuls of soyabean sauce whilst frying the rice.

Rice with Potatoes, Coriander and Mint (*Hari Chatni Pilau*)

½ teaspoon saffron threads
2 tablespoons (for saffron) plus 2 cups boiling water (for rice)

2 cups imported *basumati* rice or other uncooked long-grain white rice, washed
    and drained
½ cup clarified butter or cooking oil
4 whole cloves
One 1-inch piece of cinnamon stick
2 medium-sized boiling potatoes (about ½ pound), peeled and cut into ½-inch cubes
2 tablespoons coarsely cut fresh mint leaves
2 tablespoons scraped, finely chopped fresh ginger root
½ cup unflavored yogurt
1 teaspoon salt
¼ cup finely chopped fresh coriander
2 tablespoons finely chopped onions

Place the saffron and 2 tablespoons of the boiling water in a bowl, and soak for
10 minutes. Meanwhile, combine the rice and 3 cups of cold water in a saucepan
and bring to a boil over high heat. Stirring often, boil briskly, uncovered, for
5 minutes. Drain the rice in a sieve and set aside.

In a heavy 4-quart casserole, heat 4 tablespoons of the clarified butter over
moderate heat. Add the cloves and cinnamon and stir for 30 seconds, then add
the potatoes and, turning them constantly, fry for 5 to 6 minutes, or until they
are golden brown.

Remove the casserole from the heat and sprinkle the potatoes with the mint and
1 tablespoon of the ginger. Spread half the rice on top, smoothing it flat. Combine
the yogurt and salt with the saffron and its soaking liquid, and pour half of it
over the rice. Sprinkle the yogurt-covered rice with the remaining 1 tablespoon of
ginger, the coriander and onions, then spread the rest of the rice over the top and
pour in the remaining yogurt mixture.

Carefully and slowly pour the rest of the clarified butter and the remaining
2 cups of boiling water down the sides of the casserole. Bring to a boil, cover
tightly, and cook over high heat for 15 minutes, or until the rice is tender and
has absorbed all the liquid in the casserole.

To unmold and serve the rice, run a long, sharp knife around the inside edges
of the casserole. Place a heated serving plate upside down over the casserole and,
grasping plate and casserole firmly together, invert them. Rap the plate on a
table and the rice should slide out easily. Serve immediately.

Serves 6

Chinese Egg Fried Rice (*Tan Ch'ao Fan*)

3 tablespoons peanut or corn oil
2 tablespoons chopped scallion
3 cups leftover cooked rice
1 large egg
Salt to taste

Heat a wok or pan until very hot. Add 2 tablespoons of the oil and the chopped
scallion and stir-fry for a few seconds, then add the cooked rice (separate the

grains when rice is cold). Stir-fry until the rice is hot, about 2 minutes. Push the rice to the side, making a well in the center. Add the remaining 1 tablespoon oil. Break the egg into the center and scramble it with the oil until it has a soft consistency, then mix into the rice. Add the salt and mix well. Serve hot.

   Serves 2

Variations: Cooked vegetables, such as green beans, peas, snow peapods, vegetable steaks, chopped lettuce, and chopped spinach may be added to the rice. Add salt and monosodium glutamate to taste.

BREAD

Consumption of wholewheat bread is highly recommended for natural diet believers. Although most of us buy bread from the store, recipes for special Indian wholewheat breads are given below for those who wish to bake their own bread, especially to eat with Indian vegetable curries.

Indian Wholewheat Bread (*Chapati*)

Ingredients for the dough:

   8 ounces wholewheat flour
   ¾ to 1 cup water

Ingredients for rolling:

   2 ounces wholewheat flour

For the dough: Take 8 ounces wholewheat flour in pan. Pour ½ cup of water (excess water makes the dough sticky) and mix into a soft dough.

   Knead for 15 minutes, gradually adding the remaining water and alternately pressing and folding the dough. Sprinkle 1 or 2 tablespoonfuls water on the kneaded dough, cover with a wet cloth and leave it to swell for about half an hour. Knead the dough again for 10 minutes, moistening the fingers if it is sticky. Good results can only be obtained if the dough is kneaded sufficiently and properly.

For the bread (*chapati*):   Divide the dough into 10 to 12 pieces and using a little dry wholewheat flour shape them into round spheres. Flatten each part by placing it on the left palm and pressing it with the fingers of the right hand. Place it on a floured board and roll out with a rolling pin into a thin pancake-like form about 5 inches in diameter. Heat the griddle, rub a little grease over it to prevent the chapati from sticking and transfer the rolled chapati (pancake) on to it. Cook on medium heat. When one side dries up and tiny bubbles begin to appear, turn it over and cook till brown spots form on the surface. Press lightly around the edge with a folded cloth till it swells into a shape similar to that of two saucers inverted over each other.

Remove from the hot griddle, and apply a little butter over one side. Serve immediately. If the chapaties or bread are made in advance they should be placed one above the other, wrapped in an aluminum foil or a napkin, and stored in a container. It is, however, preferable to serve the bread immediately after preparation as they become flat and soggy on keeping.

Shallow Fried Wholewheat Bread (*Parautha*)

Ingredients:

> **10 ounces wholewheat flour**
> **A pinch of salt**
> **³/₄ to 1 cup water**
> **2 to 3 ounces clarified butter or cooking oil**

For the preparation of the dough: The same as described for the chapati or wholewheat bread.

For the Parautha: Divide the dough into 6 equal parts and shape them into round balls. Flatten and roll out each of the rounds into a flat cake about 5 inches in diameter. Coat the upper surface with a teaspoonful of clarified butter or cooking oil and fold it over into a semi-circle. Spread a little more butter over the upper surface and double-fold it lengthwise. Press it gently with the fingers, stretch a little and make it into a cone-shaped spiral, keeping the folds on the outer side, press it down so as to form a flattened ball and roll out into a *parautha*, about 5 inches in diameter. Heat griddle on a low heat, apply a little oil and transfer the *parautha* on to it. Turn it over when the under surface is lightly cooked and crisp; coat with a little butter and fry till it is crisp and golden brown on both sides.
   Serve immediately as it tends to lose crispness if stored.

Shallow Fried Wholewheat Bread with Mashed Potatoes (*Parautha Aluwala*)

Ingredients for the stuffing:

> **8 ounces boiled potatoes**
> **1 ounce finely-cut onion**
> **1 tablespoonful finely-chopped coriander leaves**
> **¹/₂ teaspoonful red pepper**
> **1 teaspoonful dried coriander seeds**
> **1 ounce clarified butter or cooking oil**
> **2 finely-cut green pepper**
> **1 teaspoonful salt**
> **¹/₂ teaspoonful allspice** *(garam masala)*
> **1 teaspoonful pomegranate seeds (optional)**
> **2 teaspoonfuls lime or lemon juice or 2 teaspoonfuls ground dried green mango**
>   **(optional)**

Ingredients for the *parautha*:

10 ounces wholewheat flour
$\frac{1}{2}$ teaspoonful salt
$\frac{3}{4}$ to 1 cup water
2 to 3 ounces clarified butter or cooking oil

For the stuffing: Boil the potatoes, cool, peel and mash them. Heat the oil and lightly fry the onion; add mashed potatoes, green pepper, coriander seeds, fresh coriander leaves, salt, red pepper, allspice, dried pomegranate seeds, and the lemon juice or powdered dried green mango. Stir for 3 to 4 minutes. Remove from the heat and cool; divide into 6 equal parts. Prepare the dough as for the plain *parautha* and divide this also into the same number of parts. Shape each part of the dough into a round ball, flatten and place on it one part of the stuffing. Round off, roll and fry as described under the plain (*parautha*) shallow fried wholewheat bread.

Indian Deep Fried Bread (*Puri*)

Ingredients for the dough:

4 ounces all purpose and 4 ounces wholewheat flour
About $\frac{1}{2}$ to $\frac{3}{4}$ cup water
1 teaspoonful melted butter or cooking oil
A pinch of salt

Ingredients for frying:

2 cups cooking oil

Mix the all purpose flour and wholewheat flour and the salt together. Make a depression in the center of the heap thus formed and pour in the water. Mix into a stiff but pliable dough and using a little melted butter, knead for about 10 to 15 minutes. Leave it covered with a wet cloth for 20 to 30 minutes. Divide the dough into 16 equal parts and shape them into round spheres. Lightly grease the rolling pin and the board with cooking oil and roll out each sphere into a thin pancake about $3\frac{1}{2}$ inches in diameter. Heat the cooking oil to smoking point and drop the rolled pancakes gently into it. Turn over immediately and press with a perforated wire, frying each slice till it swells up and acquires a light brown color. Remove from the oil and drain on a paper.

BEVERAGES

Fat free milk is the best nutritional drink. Soymilk and beverages containing soybeans are good substitutes for those who are vegans.

High-Protein Drink for Vegetarians

    2 cups skim milk
    1 ounce nonfat dry milk powder (about 5 tablespoons)
    1 banana, ripe (or 1 cup any other fresh fruit)
    2 tablespoons cocoa or carob powder
    2 tablespoons nutritional yeast
    ½ teaspoon vanilla extract

Combine all ingredients in blender.
    Makes 3 cups

Butter Milk (*Lassi*)

    2 tablespoons plain yogurt
    8 ounces glass of water
    ¼ teaspoon lemon juice
    Dash of salt
    Dash of Pepper
    Dash of coriander

Combine ingredients and add ice cubes.
    Serves 1

Fruitshake

    2 bananas, ripe
    3 cups orange juice

Combine in blender. Drink as is or freeze and use as ice cream substitute.
    Makes about 4 cups

Soy Milk

Recipe No. 1

    1 cup soy flour
    4 cups water

Mix water and soy flour. Let stand at room temperature for a couple of hours. As it sticks easily, cook soymilk in a double-boiler for about 45 minutes. Or cook in a large pot, stirring constantly. For a smoother soy milk, strain through a cheesecloth.
    Pour into quart jar and cool in refrigerator.

Recipe No. 2

To make tasty soymilk crush the beans in very hot water 180° F. (80° C.) or over. This method, which was developed by Dr. Malcolm Bourne of Cornell University, inactivates the enzyme lipoxidase, which is responsible for the bitter, beany flavor of soybeans.

Soak 1 cup of soybeans in a pot for up to 16 hours in cold water. The soaked soybeans should fill approximately 2½ cups. Discard soaking water.

Drain water from pot and put beans in blender. Add 4 cups boiling water. Blend for 2–3 minutes. It will help to keep temperature over 180° F. (80° C.), if you insulate the blender with newspapers. If the top of your blender is plastic, protect it by covering the inside with aluminum foil. If volume of soybean and water is too much, blend half at a time. Filter blended soybeans through towel. Squeeze towel thoroughly to extract all of the liquid possible. You should now have about 4 cups of liquid. Cook uncovered for 30 to 40 minutes, stirring frequently to avoid formation of skim.

Refrigerate immediately. Soymilk will keep up to five days in the refrigerator.

High-protein Drink for Vegans

> 2 cups fortified soymilk (store-bought or above recipe)
> 1 ounce soymilk powder (about 5–6 tablespoons)
> 1 banana, ripe (or 1 cup any other fresh fruit)
> 2 tablespoons cocoa or carob powder
> 4 tablespoons nutritional yeast
> ½ teaspoon vanilla extract

Combine all ingredients in blender.
Makes about 3 cups

Sesame Soymilk

This formula takes advantage of all the nutrients of soymilk, complemented by the high calcium content of the sesame seed. And since soy and sesame are complementary proteins, their combination yields an abundance of high-quality protein, making it ideal for babies, growing children, and nursing mothers.

> 1 cup soymilk, warm (see recipe or buy from store)
> 1 to 2 tablespoons *tahini* (sesame seed butter)
> Honey or molasses to taste

Combine all ingredients and mix well.

FRUITS AND DESSERTS

Fresh fruits of various kinds, consumed in their season, make the best dessert of all time. Desserts high in sugar and fatty creams may only be consumed occasionally.

Banana Grape Cup

$\frac{1}{2}$ sliced banana
6 seedless green grapes
$\frac{1}{4}$ cup orange juice
Dash of nutmeg

Combine the sliced banana and the grapes in a dessert dish. Pour the orange juice over the fruit and sprinkle with nutmeg. Chill the fruits until they are ready to serve.
Serves 1

Yogurt Sherbet and Pops

$1\frac{1}{2}$ cups yogurt
1 small canned frozen concentrated fruit juice
2 teaspoons vanilla (optional)
1 banana, ripe

Combine all ingredients. Mix well and put in tray or ice pop molds in freezer.

Peach Melba

1 pint nonfat yogurt
1 teaspoon vanilla extract
1 cup fresh black or red raspberries, or frozen, without sugar
1 tablespoon undiluted frozen apple juice concentrate, thawed
6 canned peach halves, water-packed, drained

Combine the yogurt and the vanilla. Purée the raspberries in electric blender; add $\frac{1}{4}$ cup of the purée to the yogurt, mixing well. Freeze the yogurt mixture for several hours. Add the apple juice concentrate to the remaining purée and process it again until it is smooth. Chill the peaches until they are ready to serve. When chilled, place a peach half in each of 6 dessert compotes. Top with a scoop of frozen yogurt. Spoon the raspberry sauce over all.
Serves 6

Applesauce Soufflé

1 cup unsweetened pineapple juice
2 envelopes unflavored gelatin
1 cup skim milk

1 tablespoon cornstarch
1 teaspoon almond extract
1½ cups applesauce, unsweetened
2 egg whites

Pour the pineapple juice into a small saucepan and stir in the gelatin, mixing until dissolved. Heat this to the boiling point, stirring constantly. Cool. Meanwhile, combine the milk, cornstarch, and almond extract in another saucepan; cook and stir until the mixture comes to a boil and is thickened. Stir the applesauce into the milk mixture. Add the gelatin mixture. Chill for 1 hour. Then beat the egg whites until stiff peakes form; fold them carefully into the applesauce mixture, taking care not to break the bubbles of the whites. Spoon all into a soufflé dish that has a 2-inch wax paper extension around the top of the dish. Chill for several hours. Remove the wax paper.
  Serves 6 to 8

Orange Cream

1 envelope unflavored gelatin
½ cup orange juice
1 8-ounce canned mandarin oranges, water-packed
2 cups plain nonfat yogurt
½ teaspoon ground nutmeg

Put the gelatin into a small saucepan. Add the orange juice and mix until dissolved. Add the juice from the can of oranges. Cook this mixture until the gelatin is completely dissolved. Cool the mixture. Then stir in the orange segments (reserving a few for garnishing) and the yogurt. Mix well. Pour the cream into 4 parfait glasses. Garnish each glass with the reserved orange segments. Sprinkle with mutmeg. Chill for several hours.
  Serves 4

Orange-Pineapple Sherbet

1 6-ounce canned frozen orange juice
1 6-ounce canned frozen pineapple juice
3½ cups cold water
2 tablespoons undiluted frozen apple juice concentrated, thawed
1 cup nonfat dry milk

Put all the ingredients into a large mixing bowl and beat just enough to blend everything thoroughly. Pour the mixture into ice-cube trays; freeze for 1 or 2 hours until half-frozen. Remove the sherbet to a large chilled mixing bowl; with an electric mixer beat the sherbet on low speed until the mixture is softened, then beat on high speed for 3 to 5 minutes until it is creamy but not liquid. Pour the sherbet into freezer containers or ice-cube trays. Freeze the sherbet until it is ready to serve, several hours.
  Serves 12 to 14

Chocolate Chip Cookies

> 1 cup flour
> 6 tablespoons brown sugar
> 6 tablespoons sugar
> $\frac{1}{2}$ teaspoon salt
> $\frac{1}{2}$ teaspoon baking soda
> $\frac{1}{2}$ cup margarine
> 1 teaspoon vanilla
> $\frac{1}{2}$ cup chopped nuts
> 1 cup chocolate chips
> $\frac{1}{4}$ teaspoon water
> 1 egg

Combine dry ingredients. Beat in egg. Add vanilla, morsels, and nuts. Bake 8–12 minutes at 350° F. (180° C.).

(Believe it or not—the recipe is adopted from R. F. Schlief and P. C. Wensink. *Practical Methods in Molecular Biology*. Springer-Verlag, 1981.)

Sweet Carrot Dessert (*Gajar Halva*)

> 6 medium-sized carrots (about 1 pound), scraped and coarsely grated
> 1 quart milk
> 1 cup light cream
> 1 cup jaggery (raw cane sugar), or substitute dark-brown sugar combined with dark molasses
> $\frac{1}{2}$ cup sugar
> $1\frac{1}{2}$ cups whole blanched almonds (about 8 ounces), pulverized in a blender or with a nut grinder
> $\frac{1}{4}$ cup clarified unsalted butter
> The seeds of 10 cardamom pods or $\frac{1}{2}$ teaspoon cardamom seeds, wrapped in a kitchen towel and crushed with a rolling pin
> $\frac{1}{4}$ cup unsalted pistachios, toasted
> $\frac{1}{4}$ cup unsalted, slivered blanched almonds, toasted

In a deep heavy saucepan, combine the carrots, milk and cream. Stirring constantly, bring to a boil over high heat. Reduce the heat to moderate and, stirring occasionally, cook for 1 hour, or until the mixture has reduced to about half its original volume and is thick enough to coat a spoon heavily. Stir in the jaggery (or brown sugar and molasses) and the sugar, and continue cooking for 10 minutes. Reduce the heat to lowest possible point, add the pulverized almonds and the clarified butter, and stir for 10 minutes more, or until the halva mixture is thick enough to draw away from the sides and bottom of the pan in solid mass. Remove the pan from the heat and stir in the cardamom.

With a metal spatula, spread the halva on a large heat proof platter, mound it slightly in the center, and decorate the top with pistachios and slivered almonds. Serve warm or at room temperature.

Serves 6 to 8

Milk and Rice Pudding with Cardamom and Nuts (*Khir*)

2 quarts milk
$\frac{1}{3}$ cup imported *basumati* rice or other uncooked long-grain white rice, washed
    and drained
1 cup sugar
$\frac{1}{2}$ cup finely chopped unsalted blanched almonds
The seeds of 3 whole cardamom pods or $\frac{1}{4}$ teaspoon cardamom seeds, coarsely
    crushed in a mortar and pestle or in a bowl with the back of a spoon
1 teaspoon rose water
$\frac{1}{4}$ cup unsalted sliced, blanched almonds, lightly toasted

In a heavy saucepan, bring the milk to a boil over high heat, stirring constantly
to prevent a skin forming on the surface. Reduce the heat to moderate and,
stirring occasionally, cook for 30 minutes. Add the rice and continue cooking and
stirring frequently for 30 minutes, or until the rice is very soft, in fect until the
grains have almost disintegrated.

Add the sugar and finely chopped almonds and stir for 15 minutes over low
heat until the pudding is thick enough to coat the spoon heavily. Remove the pan
from the heat, stir in the cardamom and rose water, and pour the pudding into a
shallow 7-by-12-inch baking dish. With a rubber spatula spread it out evenly
and smooth the top. Then sprinkle with the toasted almonds. Refrigerate the *khir*
for at least 4 hours, or until it is thoroughly chilled and somewhat firm to the touch.
    Serves 10 to 12

MISCELLANEOUS

Bean Burgers

You can make these in quantity and freeze them for future use. Soybeans or any
kind of beans plus oatmeal can be used as the base of bean burgers.

1 cup raw beans
1 cup uncooked oatmeal
$\frac{1}{2}$ cup nutritional yeast
$\frac{1}{2}$ teaspoon garlic powder
1 teaspoon dry mustard
1 teaspoon chilli powder
1 teaspoon onion powder
2 tablespoons vegetable oil

Cook beans, mash, and combine with oatmeal, yeast, garlic, mustard chilli, and
onion powder. Heat in oven for a few minutes at 300° F. (150° C.). (This inhibits
soaking up oil during sautéing.) Form into six thin burgers and fry in oil over low
heat. Top with sliced onion and catsup and serve on bread or bun.
    Makes 6 servings

Vegetable Casserole

This recipe calls for one large or two small casserole dishes.

> 2 medium onion, boiled
> 3 large or 4 medium potatoes
> 10-ounce packet frozen cauliflower
> 10-ounce packet frozen string beans
> 10-ounce packet frozen peas
> 1 canned condensed soup-cream type such a mushroom, celery or asparagus
> ½ cup nutritional yeast
> 1 large tomato, sliced thin

Preheat onions in 300° F. (150° C.) oven for a few minutes and then sauté in oil until slightly brown. Boil vegetables and potatoes until they are almost—but not quite—soft. Reserve vegetable cooking water. Combine onions, potatoes, vegetables, and soup in large bowl, adding about 1 cup of vegetable stock. Cover with sliced tomato, top with yeast, and bake in 350° F. (180° C.) oven for 10 minutes or until yeast begins to brown.

Makes 6 servings

Soybean Casserole

> 3 tablespoons vegetable oil
> 1 medium onion, chopped
> 1 clove garlic, chopped
> ½ green pepper, chopped
> 3 cups cooked soybeans
> ½ cup tomato sauce
> 1 teaspoon salt
> ½ cup bread crumbs
> 4 ounces cheddar cheese, grated
> 3 tablespoons sesame seeds
> Preheat oven to 375° F. (190° C.)

Heat oil in large skillet. Sauté onion, garlic, and green pepper. Add soybeans, tomato sauce, salt, and bread crumbs, and mix. Transfer mixture into an oiled casserole dish. Sprinkle cheese on top, and then sesame seeds.

Cover and bake for 20 minutes or until cheese is melted.

Savory Patties

> ⅔ cup dry soybeans
> 3 cups water
> 1¼ cups water
> 1 teaspoon onion powder or 1 chopped onion
> 1 teaspoon Italian seasoning
> 2 tablespoons soy sauce
> ½ teaspoon salt

1⅓ cups rolled oats
2 tablespoons oil

Soak the soybeans overnight in 3 cups water, then drain (yields 2 cups soaked beans). Grind the soybeans or blend in 1¼ cups water until the texture becomes quite fine. Add the seasonings and the rolled oats. Allow the mixture to stand 10 minutes until oats absorb the liquid. Stir again and drop by rounded table-spoon into a lightly oiled skillet over moderate heat (350° F. or 180° C. in an electric skillet). Cover and cook the patties for about 10 minutes or until brown. Turn, cover, and cook until browned. Reduce the heat and allow the patties to cook 10 minutes longer. Serve with tomato sauce (see the recipe below).

   Makes 16 patties, 2 per serving

Tomato Sauce

   1 large onion, finely chopped
   1 tablespoon oil
   2 cans condensed tomato soup (undiluted)
   ½ teaspoon oregano or basil

Sauté the onion in the oil over a very low heat; do not brown. Add the tomato soup and oregano or basil. Heat the sauce until bubbly and serve on warm Savory Patties.

Potato Kugel

   6 medium raw potatoes
   2–3 raw carrots
   1 large onion
   1 clove garlic, minced
   2 eggs, beaten
   3 tablespoons oil
   2 teaspoons salt
   ¼ cup whole-grain or enriched bread crumbs
   ¾ cup dry skim-milk powder
   Topping, if desired: 1 cup grated cheese

Grate the potatoes, carrots, and onion into a large bowl. Drain off the accumu-lated liquid. Stir in the remaining ingredients, adding the milk powder slowly to avoid lumps. Spread mixture in an oiled 7×7-inch pan and bake at 350° F. (180°C.) for 45 minutes to 1 hour. The kugel is done when the edges are brown and a knife inserted in center of the kugel comes out dry. If desired, add the grated cheese on top of the kugel at this point and leave in the oven 5 minutes longer.

   Makes 8 servings

Eggplant Parmigiana (*Parmigiana di Melanzane*)

   1 eggplant, about 1 pound
   ¼ cup wheat germ or bread crumbs

2 eggs
4 tablespoons flour
4 tablespoons oil
1 canned tomato sauce (15 ounces)
½ cup onions, minced
1 clove garlic, minced
2 teaspoons oregano
⅛ teaspoon basil
⅛ teaspoon pepper
½ pound mozzarella cheese, sliced thin
1 cup grated parmesan cheese

Peel eggplant and cut into ½ inch-thick slices. Warm slices in 300° F. (150° C.) oven for a few minutes. Beat eggs with fork and mix in wheat germ. Dip slices of eggplant in flour and then in wheat germ-egg mixture and once again in flour. Sauté in oil over medium-low heat until brown and crisp on both sides. Combine tomato sauce and flavorings in saucepan. Bring to boil and then simmer for 20 minutes. Place slices of eggplant in roasting pan, cover with mozzarella cheese, followed by tomato sauce, and top with parmesan cheese. Bake at 400° F. (200° C.) for 15 minutes. Makes 6 servings.

Mushroom Omelette

2 cups mushrooms, sliced
4 tablespoons onions, chopped
3 tablespoons butter or margarine
6 eggs, room temperature
⅛ teaspoon pepper

Preheat mushrooms and onions in 300° F. (150° C.) oven for a few minutes. Melt 2 tablespoons butter or margarine in large frying pan. Add mushrooms and onions and sauté until brown.

In separate large frying pan—preferably one with sloping sides—melt 1 tablespoon butter or margarine. Beat eggs, add 3 tablespoons water. Pour eggs into pan, stirring the surface with a fork. Allow edges to congeal—about 30 seconds—and then, tilting the pan slightly, coax the liquid egg on top to the edge of the pan and under the congealed part of the omelette. After no liquid is left on top, add mushrooms, slide omelette onto plate . Fold, divide in three parts, and serve.

Makes 3 servings

Mushroom Quiche

1 pound mushrooms, chopped
1 cup onions, chopped
½ teaspoon ginger
4 teaspoons oil
3 teaspoons red wine
4 eggs, beaten

1 store-bought piecrust stick
½ pint heavy cream
4 ounces cheddar or Gruyere cheese, sliced thin

Warm mushrooms and onions in 300° F. (150° C.) oven for a few minutes. Add ginger and sauté in oil and wine for about 10 minutes in saucepan. Make piecrust according to directions on package, using a deep dish suitable for baking (capacity should be at least 1½ quarts). Gradually add eggs and cream to saucepan, stirring continuously. Pour into piecrust shell and top with cheese. Bake 35 minutes at 350° F. (180° C.). Makes about 8 servings.

Wheat Tortillas with filling

1 cup dry pinto beans
1 canned tomato soup
1 teaspoon onion salt
3 cups wholewheat flour
1 teaspoon salt
⅓ cup oil
1 cup water
6–8 tablespoons chopped parsley
6–8 leaves salad greens (e.g., cabbage, lettuce), shredded
5–6 green onions (scallions) with tops, sliced

To make the filling: Soak the pinto beans overnight in water to cover. Drain. Cook the beans in fresh water until they are tender. Drain again. Add the tomato soup and onion salt to the beans and cook the mixture while preparing the tortillas.

To make tortillas: Mix the flour with the salt. In a separate bowl, combine the oil and water and beat together with a fork. Stir the oil-water mixture into the flour, wetting the flour as evenly as possible. Mix. Divide the dough into 12 parts. Roll or pat each piece of dough into a thin circle of about 5 inches in diameter. Cook the tortillas on an ungreased skillet or on a grill.

Wholewheat Quick Pizza

2 cups wholewheat flour
1 package (1 tablespoon) active dry yeast
¾ teaspoon salt
1 cup hot tap water
1 tablespoon cooking oil
1 teaspoon honey

Pour flour into a large mixing bowl. Add yeast and salt to flour and stir to blend. Add rest of the ingredients to flour mixture and beat vigorously until well mixed. Cover with plastic wrap and place in a warm spot for 10 minutes. Punch down and place dough in a greased 14-inch pizza pan. Press with fingers to evenly cover bottom pan and up the sides to form a rim. Preheat oven to 425° F. (220° C.).

Ingredients for topping:

> 2 cups tomato sauce
> 1 cup sliced mushrooms, sautéed
> ½ cup sliced onions, sautéed
> ½ cup sliced, pitted ripe olives
> ½ teaspoon crumbled oregano
> ½ teaspoon crumbled basil
> 6 ounces mozzarella cheese, shredded or sliced
> ¼ cup freshly grated parmesan cheese; olive oil

Spread sauce on dough, distribute remaining ingredients evenly over the top, ending with a sprinkling of olive oil. Bake at 425° F. (220° C.) for 15 to 20 minutes until crust is golden brown and cheese is melted. You can vary the topping according to your taste.

Variation: Here's another topping that's extra crispy and features flavorful almonds:

> 1 teaspoon oil
> 1 cup shredded mozzarella cheese
> 2 medium tomatoes, thinly sliced
> ¾ cup sliced mushrooms
> 2 tablespoons sliced green onion
> 1 teaspoon mixed basil and oregano
> ¼ teaspoon thyme
> ¼ cup slivered almonds
> 1 tablespoon freshly grated parmesan cheese

Brush oil on prepared pizza dough and sprinkle mozzarella cheese evenly over the surface. Top with remaining ingredients in given order, ending with the parmesan. Bake on the lowest rack of a 400° F. (205° C.) oven until crust is browned and cheese is melted and bubbling. Remove from oven.

Before serving sprinkle top of pie with 1 tablespoon chopped parsley and cut in wedges to serve.

Pancake Delight

> 1 cup buckwheat flour
> 1 cup wholewheat flour
> 2 teaspoons baking powder
> ½ teaspoon baking soda
> ¼ teaspoon salt (optional)
> ¼ teaspoon caraway seeds
> ¼ teaspoon turmeric
> ¼ teaspoon curry

¼ teaspoon powdered allspice
⅛ teaspoon celery seeds
¼ teaspoon onion salt
2 cups buttermilk

Place the flours, baking powder, baking soda, salt, spices, and onion salt in a large bowl. Add the butter-milk, stirring lightly until the mixture is well blended. Pour some of the mixture onto a lightly greased griddle or frying pan. Cook until pancakes are golden brown underneath. Turn once.

Makes 16 pancakes

Crepes

1 cup wholewheat pastry flour
1¼ cups skim milk
4 egg whites, stiffly beaten

Blend the milk with the flour until smooth, then carefully fold in the stiffly beaten egg whites. Heat a medium-sized nonstick skillet until very hot. Then pour in a scant ¼ cup batter, rotating the pan to cover the bottom and to distribute the batter evenly. Brown the crepe on both sides until golden brown.

Crepes are a versatile dish for any meal, with fillings ranging from cheese to Chinese vegetables, fruits, meat and fish.

Ratatouille Crepes

1 onion sliced
3 medium zucchini, sliced
2 medium crookneck squash, sliced
10 mushrooms sliced
1 green pepper, cut into strips
1 clove garlic, minced
1 6-ounce canned tomato paste
2 tablespoons chopped pimientos
1 teaspoon Italian herb seasoning
¼ teaspoon pepper
14 to 16 premade crepes
Chopped parsley, to garnish

In a heated nonstick skillet, add the onions to brown. Stir constantly over a medium flame to prevent scorching. Then add a few tablespoons of water, bring to a boil, and add the other vegetables, cooking until the vegetables are almost limp. Stir in a tomato paste, 1 can of water, pimiento, and seasoning. Simmer for 10 to 15 minutes.

Place about 3 tablespoons of vegetable mixture on each crepe; fold the sides to overlap. Place the crepes on serving plates, allowing 2 per person. Spoon the remaining mixture over the folded crepes. Garnish with chopped parsley. Serves 8.

Example of Nutritionally Balanced Vegetarian Menus

The menus 1 to 4 are devised by the New York City Department of Health's Bureau of Nutrition. Menus 1, 2 are for ovolacto- and 3, 4, for lacto-vegetarians. These are designed to provide adequate protein and the daily requirements of vitamins and minerals without overloading on saturated fats, cholesterol, and calories. The average Calorie supply is about 2,400 daily. The menus 5 and 6 are devised by the Department of Nutrition of the School of Health at Loma Linda University, California. These provide 2,800 to 2,900 Calories a day and about 80 grams of protein each. To find your individual needs consult section "Determining Proper Calorie Intake" in Chapter 4. "Adjust calories by changing portion size or cut down on fats, if you need to reduce calories. The recipes for the starred items are given in Appendix A on "Natural Diet Recipes."

SAMPLE MENU 1

BREAKFAST:

Cantaloupe	½ medium
Shredded-wheat biscuits	2
Whole-grain or enriched toast	1 slice
Margarine	1 pat (1 teaspoon)
Skim milk	1 cup

LUNCH:

Vegetable Juice	1 cup
Egg-salad sandwich:	1
2 slices whole-grain bread	
1 medium egg	
1 tablespoon diced celery	
1 teaspoon mayonnaise	
Pear	1 medium

SNACKS:

Dried apricot halves	4
Almonds	¼ cup

DINNER:

Soy and brown-rice loaf*	1 cup
carrots	½ cup
Broccoli	½ cup
Margarine	1 pat
Waldorf Salad:	6 oz
½ cup diced apple	
1 tablespoon diced celery	
1 tablespoon raisins	
1 tablespoon chopped walnuts	
1 tablespoon mayonnaise	
Vanilla pudding	½ cup

SANCK:

Buttermilk or yogurt	1 cup
Graham crackers	4

SAMPLE MENU 2

BREAKFAST:

Grapefruit	½
Sliced cheese	1 oz
Whole-grain or enriched toast	2 slices
Margarine	1 pat
Skim milk	½ cup

LUNCH:

Black beans and rice	1 cup
Mixed green salad	
Cottage cheese	½ cup
Salad dressing	1 tablespoon
Whole-grain or enriched bread	1 slice
Margarine	1 pat
Cantaloupe	1 slice

SNACK:

Yogurt	1 cup
Sunflower seeds	¼ cup

DINNER:

Potato kugel*	1 cup
Baked acorn squash	½

Coleslaw	½ cup
Mayonnaise	1 teaspoon
Whole-grain or enriched bread	1 slice
Margarine	1 pat
Pear	1 medium

SNACK:

Milk	½ cup
Bulgur wheat	¾ cup
Raisins	¼ cup

SAMPLE MENU 3

BREAKFAST:

Grapefruit juice	½ cup
Oatmeal	1 cup
Whole-grain or enriched toast	1 slice
Margarine	1 pat
Skim milk	½ cup

SNACK:

| Yogurt | ½ cup |
| Sesame bread sticks | 4–6 |

LUNCH:

Grilled cheese sandwich:	1
2 slices whole-grain toast	
1 ounce cheese	
1 pat margarine	
Tossed green salad	
Salad dressing	1 tablespoon
Fresh fruit	1 cup

SNACK:

| Raisins | ¼ cup |
| Peanuts | ¼ cup |

DINNER:

Tomato juice	½ cup
Mixed bean salad*	1 cup
Pancake delight*	
Apple	1 medium

SNACK:

Whole-grain or enriched cereal	1 cup
Milk	½ cup

SAMPLE MENU 4

BREAKFAST:

Orange	1 medium
Cottage cheese	¼ cup
Whole-grain or enriched toast	2 slices
Margarine	1 pat
Skim milk	½ cup

SNACK:

Part-skimmed cheese	1 slice
Whole-grain or enriched crackers	4–6

LUNCH:

Split-pea soup	1 cup
Sesame crackers*	
Tomato and cucumber salad	
Salad dressing	1 tablespoon
Baked apple	
Skim milk	½ cup

SNACK:

Prunes	2
Roasted soybeans	¼ cup

DINNER:

Fresh fruit	1 cup
Baked macaroni and cheese	1 cup
Collard greens	½ cup
Whole-grain or enriched bread	1 slice
Margarine	2 pats
Junket	½ cup

SNACK:

Whole-grain or enriched roll	1
Buttermilk	½ cup

SAMPLE MENU 5

BREAKFAST:

Orange	1
Oatmeal (⅔ cup dry) with	
1 tablespoon molasses	
¼ cup raisins	
⅔ cup nondairy creamer or powdered soy milk	
Whole-wheat toast	2 slices
Margarine	2 pats
Peanut butter	1 tablespoon

LUNCH:

Savory patties*	2 servings
Baked potato	1
Margarine	1 tablespoon
Cooked turnip greens	1 cup
Large tomato, sliced	1
Whole-wheat bread	1 slice
Margarine	1 teaspoon

DINNER:

Wheat tortillas with filling*	2 servings
Apple	1 medium
Figs	5 large dried
Raw almonds	15

SAMPLE MENU 6

BREAKFAST:

Orange	1
Whole-wheat cooked cereal, 1 cup with	
1 tablespoon molasses	
¼ cup raisins	
⅓ cup nondairy creamer or powdered soy milk	
Banana	1
Whole-wheat toast	2 slices
Margarine	2 teaspoons
Peanut butter	2 tablespoons

LUNCH:

Black beans on rice*	2 servings
Diced carrots, cooked	½ cup
or	
Summer squash, diced	1 cup
Coleslaw	⅔ cup
Date bread	2 slices

SUPPER:

Thick vegetable soup*	2 servings
Kale (no stems), cooked	¾ cup
Whole-wheat bread	1 slice
Margarine	1 pat

Example of Nutritionally and Calorically Balanced Non-Vegetarian Diet for a Week

These menus are essentially followed from those of Jelia Witschi of Harvard University. The wide variety of foods furnish adequate protein, minerals and vitamins for nutritionally balanced meals. The average Calorie supply is about 1,500 per day—a weight maintenance program for a typical 100–pound moderately active woman. To find your individual needs, consult section "Determining Proper Calorie Intake" in Chapter 4.

SUNDAY

BREAKFAST:

Blueberries (fresh or unsweetened)	½ cup
Cornflakes	¾ cup
Toast	1 slice
Margarine	1 tsp
Skim or low fat milk	1 cup

SNACK:

Orange	1 med.

LUNCH:

Broiled hamburger patty	2 oz
Hamburger roll	1 medium
Dill pickles	
Catsup	1 tsp
Banana	1 small
Skim or low fat milk	1 cup

SNACK:

Plain yogurt	½ cup
Fresh strawberries	¼ cup

DINNER:

Hot chicken consomme with lemon slice

Filet of sole with mushrooms	3 oz.
Boiled potato and carrots with light brown sugar sauce	½ cup
Avocado-grapefruit salad served on leaves of fresh spinach	¼ of each
French dressing	1 tbsp
Margarine for cooking	1 tsp
Lemon sponge cupcake	1

SNACK:

Plain popcorn	1 cup

MONDAY

BREAKFAST:

Orange juice	½ cup
Scrambled egg in 1½ tsp margarine	1
English muffin	½
Margarine	1 tsp
Skim or low-fat milk	1 cup

SNACK:

Plain raisin toast with low calorie jelly	1 slice

LUNCH:

Sliced lean ham	2 oz
Coleslaw	1½ cup
Roll	1 small
Pineapple (fresh or unsweetened)	2 slices
Skim or low-fat milk	1 cup

SNACK:

Coffee frappe made with skim milk	½ cup
Instant coffee	1 tsp
Ice cubes	½ cup

DINNER:

Tomato soup (hot or chilled) sprinkled with basil	1 cup
Baked chicken with peach half	3 oz
Brussels sprouts and onions: brussels sprouts, ½ cup; onions	½ cup

Boiled rice	½ cup
Margarine	1 tsp
Grapes	12

SNACK:

Whole-wheat melba toast	2
Peanut butter	2 tsp

TUESDAY

BREAKFAST:

Apricot nectar	½ cup
Melted cheese on toast	1 slice
Skim or low-fat milk	1 cup

SNACK:

Sliced banana with sour cream
  ½ banana with 1 tbsp sour cream

LUNCH:

Tuna-stuffed tomato on lettuce	
2 oz tuna: 1 med. tomato	
French dressing	1 tbsp
Wheat thins	10
Lemon cake pudding	½ cup
Skim or low-fat milk	1 cup

SANACK:

Graham crackers	2

DINNER:

Cream of mushroom soup	1 cup
(Mushroom, onions, broth, skim milk)	
London broil	3 oz
Baked winter squash	½ cup
Margarine	1 tsp
Spinach salad	1 cup
Italian dressing	1 tbsp
Cantaloupe with lime wedge	¼

SNACK:

Raisins	3 tbsp

WEDNESDAY

BREAKFAST:

Orange grapefruit juice	½ cup
Crispy grilled Canadian bacon	1 slice
Toast	1 slice
Margarine	1 tsp
Skim or low-fat milk	1 cup

SNACK:

Apple	1 small

LUNCH:

Grilled frankfurter	1
Frankfutrter roll	1
Potato salad	½ cup
Pear (fresh or unsweetened)	1 small
Skim or low-fat milk	1 cup

SNACK:

Almonds	8

DINNER:

Jellied consomme with lemon slice	1 cup
Lamb Kabab (lamb, onion, mushrooms, tomato, green peppers)	3 oz lamb
Syrian bread or small roll	1
Green salad	
Low calorie dressing	1 tbsp
Watermelon	1 medium slice

SNACK:

Ice milk	⅓ cup

THURSDAY

BREAKFAST:

Pineapple juice	½ cup
Raisin toast	2 slices
Peanut butter	1 tbsp
Skim or low-fat milk	1 cup

SNACK:

    Hard candy   2 large

LUNCH:

Chili concorne with beans	⅔ cup
Saltines	2
Carrot and celery sticks	2 each
Orange	1 medium
Skim or low fat milk	1 cup

SNACK:

    Pimento and Neufchatel cheese on celery   1 tbsp cheese

DINNER:

Beef boullion	
Broiled veal chop (lean)	3 oz
Baked potato	1 medium
Margarine	1 tsp
Hot sliced beets with ½ tsp margarine	½ cup
Lettuce wedge with herbed wine vinegar	
Peach melba, 1 medium with ¼ cup raspberries (fresh or unsweetened)	

SNACK:

    Plain yogurt with no calorie coffee flavoring   ½ cup

FRIDAY

BREAKFAST:

Fresh strawberries	½ cup
Toasted English muffin	1
Margarine	2 tsp
Poached egg	1
Skim or low-fat milk	1 cup

SNACK:

    Plums fresh or unsweetened   2 small

LUNCH:

Tomato rice soup	
Chicken sandwich, chicken	2 oz

Bread	2 slices
Mayonnaise	1 tsp
Relish tray (cauliflowerets with green pepper served with chili sauce)	½ cup
Orange ambrosia: orange coconut, 1 tbsp	1 medium

SNACK:

Pretzel, 3 rings	5 medium

DINNER:

Jellied mushroom soup	1 cup
Grilled ham steak	3 oz
Corn on the cob	1 medium
Broccoli	½ cup
Pineapple (fresh or unsweetened) with mint	½ cup

SNACK:

Skim or low-fat milk	1 cup
Vanilla wafers	3 small

SATURDAY

BREAKFAST:

Apple juice	½ cup
Cheerios	¾ cup
Date muffin	1
Margarine	1 tsp
Skim or low-fat milk	1 cup

SNACk:

Grapefruit	½

LUNCH:

Lean corned beef sandwich:	
corned beef	2 oz
rye bread	2 slices
mustard	
Sauerkraut	½ cup
Dill pickles	
Blackberries (fresh or unsweetened)	½ cup

SNACK:

    Carrot sticks with cottage cheese and chives:
        carrot   1
        cheese   ¼

DINNER:

Cream of celery soup with skim or low-fat milk — 1 cup
Seafood creole — ¾ cup
Boiled noodles — ½ cup
Tossed salad with herbs, vinegar — 1 cup
Cantaloupe — ¼
  with lime sherbet

SNACKS:

Peanuts — 6–8

SOURCE: *Food and Fitness*, Blue Cross Association, 1973.

Caloric Values of Popular Fast Foods and Percent of Total Calories of Protein, Carbohydrate and Fat

Item	Total Calories	% Protein Calories	% Carbo-hydrate Calories	% Fat Calories
McDonald's Big Mac	541	19	29	52
Burger King Whopper	606	19	34	47
Burger Chef Hamburger	258	17	37	46
Dairy Queen Cheese Dog	330	18	29	52
Taco Bell Taco	186	32	30	38
Pizza Hut Thin 'N Crispy Cheese Pizza ($\frac{1}{2}$ of 10-inch pie)	450	22	48	30
Pizza Hut Thick 'N Chewy Pepperoni Pizza ($\frac{1}{2}$ of 10-inch pie)	560	22	49	29
Arthur Treacher's Fish Sandwich	440	15	36	49
Burger King Whaler	486	15	53	32
McDonald's Filet-O-Fish	402	15	34	51
Long John Silver's Fish (2 pieces)	318	23	23	54
Kentucky Fried Chicken Original Recipe Dinner	830	25	26	49
Kentucky Fried Chicken, extra crispy Dinner (3 pieces chicken)	950	22	27	51
McDonald's Egg McMuffin	352	20	29	51
Burger King French Fries	214	6	52	42
Arthur Treacher's Coleslaw	123	4	37	59
Dairy Queen Onion Rings	300	7	43	50
McDonald's Apple Pie	300	3	41	56
Burger King Vanilla Shake (12 oz)	332	12	59	29
McDonald's Chocolate Shake (12 oz)	364	12	66	22
Dairy Queen Bannana Split	540	8	67	25

SOURCE: Modified from data supplied by the companies to the Senate Select committee on Nutrition and Human Needs.

List of Manufacturers of Meat Analogues and of Stores That are Likely to Carry Their Products

If you have difficulty finding meat analogues in your area, the following list should be helpful. Write to the company's marketing or customer service department. These departments will also send recipe booklets upon request.

Worthington foods, a division of Miles Laboratories Inc., 900 Proprietors Road, Worthington, OH 43085. Products found in most health-food stores.

Loma Linda Foods, 11503 Pierce Street, Riverside, CA 92515. Products found in many supermarket chains and in some health-food stores.

Morningstar Farms, a division of Miles Laboratories Inc., 7123 West 65th Street, Chicago, IL 60638. Nationally distributed in supermarkets and grocery stores.

Appendix **F**

The Metric System, and Equivalent Level Measures and Weights

The metric system is a standardized system of measurement that is used internationally. However, countries such as the Unites States also employs another system of measurement based on the old English system. In the field of dietetics, both systems are used. The following chart gives equivalents for common household measures.

Equivalent Level Measures and Weights

60 drops	=1 teaspoon (tsp) 5 cubic centimeters (cc) 5 grams (g)	16 Tbsp	=1 cup 240 g 250 milliliter (ml) 8 oz (fluid) ½ pound (1b)
1 tsp	=5 g 5 cc		
		2 cups	= 1 pint 480 g 500 ml 16 oz (fluid) 1 lb
3 tsp	=1 tablespoon (tbsp) 15 cc 15 g		
1 dessert- spoon	=10 g 10 cc	4 cups	=2 pints 1 quart 1,000 or 960 cc 1,000 ml 1 kilogram (kg) 2.2 lb
2 Tbsp	=30 cc 30 g 1 ounce (oz) (fluid)		
4 Tbsp	=¼ cup 60 cc 60 g	2 pints 4 quarts 8 quarts 2 gallons 4 pecks 8 gallons	=1 quart =1 gallon = 1 peck =1 peck =1 bushel = 1 bushel
8 Tbsp	=½ cup 120 cc 120 g		

Equivalents in Grams

For easy computing purposes, the cubic centimeter (cc) or milliliter (ml) is considered equivalent to 1 gram (g):

1 cc = 1 ml	1,000 cc = 1 liter (l)
1 g	1 kg
1,000 milligram (mg)	1,000 g
1,000,000 microgram (μg)	

Also for easy computing, one ounce equals 30 g or 30 cc

1 quart	= 960 g	1 glass (8 oz) = 240 g	
1 pint	= 480 g	½ glass (4 oz) = 120 g	
1 cup	= 240 g	1 orange juice glass = 100 to 120g	
½ cup	= 120 g	1 tbsp = 15 g	
1 soup cup	= 120 g	1 tsp = 5 g	

A Guide To Approximate Storage Time for Foods

Food	Storage Conditions		
	Cool room (12°C)	Refrigerator (4°C)	Freezer (−20°C)
Apple	until ripe	not recommended	not recommended
Brassicas & leaf vegetables	1 day	5 days	6–9 months
Bacon, smoked	5–7 days	10–14 days	6 months
Bread	1–2 days	2–4 days	3 months
Butter and Margarine	3–7 days	7–14 days	1 month
Cheese, cottage	not recommended	1 week	not recommended
Cheese, hard	5–10 days	1–4 weeks	3 months
Cheese, soft	4–5 days	7–10 days	1 month
Chicken	2 days	3–4 days	10–12 months
Citrus fruit	2 weeks	2–3 weeks	3–6 weeks
Eggs	1–2 weeks	up to 4 weeks	not recommended
Eggs-Hard Boiled in Shell	1 day	5–7 days	not recommended
Fish	not recommended	1–2 days	3–6 months
Fish, cooked	not recommended	3–4 days	3–4 months
Fish, smoked	2 days	2–4 days	6–12 months
Meat, Steak	1 day	2–3 days	4 months
Meat, Ground	not recommended	2–4 days	3 months
Meat, organ (e.g. liver)	not recommended	1–2 days	3–4 months
Melons	until ripe	1 week	not recommended
Milk	1 day	3–4 days	2 months (homogenized)
Mushrooms	1 day	2–3 days	3–4 months
Oils	up to 6 months	not recommended	not recommended
Orchard fruit, e.g. pears	1–3 days	3–7 days	6–9 months
Pineapples	until ripe	10 days	not recommended
Pods and seeds e.g. beans and corn	1 day (unshelled)	1–2 days (shelled)	6–9 months
Potatoes and root vegetable	1 week	not recommended	6–9 months (carrots only)
Salad leaves	1 day	3–7 days	not recommended
Soft fruits e.g. banana	1 day	2–3 days	7–9 months (not banana)
Stalks and shoots e.g. broccoli	2–4 days	5–7 days	2 months
Tomatoes	until ripe	7–14 days	not recommended
Vegetable fruit e.g. cucumber, eggplant	2–4 days	1 week	2 months
Yogurt	not recommended	7 days	2 months (sugar added)

Bibliography*

Asher, W. L. (editor). 1974. *Treating the Obese*. Medcom Press, New York.

Åstrand, P. O. and K. Rodhl. 1970. *Textbook of Work Physiology*. McGraw-Hill Book Co., New York.

Benet, S. 1976. *How to Live to be 100: The Life-style of the People of the Caucasus*. The Dial Press, New York.

Bloomfield, H. H., M. P. Cain and D. T. Jaffe. 1975. *Transcendental Meditation*. Delacorte Press, New York.

Bray, G. A. and J. E. Bethune (editors). 1974. *Treatment and Management of Obesity*. Harper & Row, Publishers, New York.

Brewster, L. and M. F. Jacobson. 1978. *The Changing American Diet*. The Center for Science in Public Interest, Washington, D.C.

Brody, J. E. 1981. *Jane Brody's Nutrition Book*. W. W. Norton and Co., New York.

Brown, B. 1977. *Stress and the Art of Biofeedback*. Harper & Row, Publishers, New York.

Burkitt, D. 1979. *Eat Right to Stay Healthy*. Arco, New York.

Burkitt, D. and H. Trowell. 1975. *Refined Carbohydrate Foods and Disease*. Academic Press, London.

Burnet, S. F. M. 1974. *Intrinsic Mutagenesis: A Genetic Approach to Aging*. John Wiley & Sons, New York.

Caliendo, Mary A. 1981. *Nutrition and Preventive Health Care*. Macmillan Publishing Co., Inc., New York.

Calloway, D. H. and K. O. Carpenter. 1981. *Nutrition and Health*. Saunders College Publishing, Philadelphia.

Chafetz, M. 1978. *How Drinking Can be Good for You*. Stein and Day, New York.

Church, C. F. and H. N. Church. 1975. *Food Values of Portions Commonly Used*. 12th ed. J. B. Lippincott Co., Philadelphia.

Corbin, C. 1980. *Nutrition*. Holt, Rinehart and Winston, New York.

Farquhar, John W. 1978. *The American Way of Life Need Not be Hazardous to Your Health*. W. W. Norton and Co., New York.

---

* Includes selective titles. Journal articles (with few exceptions) are not included in bibliography, but are cited at appropriate places in the text. Books on recipe sources are cited in Appendix A.

258

Feingold, B. F. 1974. *Why Your Child is Hyperactive*. Random House, New York.

Fisher, S. 1973. *Body Consciousness*. Prentice-Hall, Inc., Englewood Cliffs, New Jersey.

Fomon, S. J. 1974. *Infant Nutrition*. 2nd ed. W. B. Saunders Co., Philadelphia.

Forem, J. 1973. *Transcendental Meditation, Maharishi Mahesh Yogi and the Science of Creative Intelligence*. E. P. Dutton & Co., Inc., New York.

Fort, J. 1973. *Alcohol: Out greatest Drug Problem*. McGraw-Hill Book Co., New York.

Frank, B. S. 1976. *Doctor Frank's No-Aging Diet*. The Dial Press, New York.

Freemon, F. R. 1972. *Sleep Research: A Critical Review*. Charles C. Thomas Publishers, Springfield, Illinois.

Friedman, M. and R. H. Rosenman. 1974. *Type A Behavior and Your Heart*. Alfred A. Knopf, New York.

Geist, V. 1978. *Life Strategies, Human Evolution, Environmental Design—Towards a Biological Theory of Health*. Springer-Verlag, New York.

Glass, D. C. 1977. *Stress and Coronary Prone Behavior*. Lawrence Erlbaum Associates, New York.

Goodhart, R. S. and M. E. Shils (editors). 1973. *Modern Nutrition in Health and Disease*. 5th ed. Lea and Febiger, Philadelphia.

Goodwin, M. T. 1974. *Better Living Through Better Eating*. 2nd ed. Montgomery County Health Department, Rockville, Maryland.

Gordon, P. 1974. *Free Radicals and the Aging Process. In: Theoretical Aspects of Aging*, M. Rockstein, editor. Academic Press, New York.

Gormican, A. 1971. *Controlling Diabetes with Diet*. Charles C. Thomas Publishers, Springfield, Illinois.

Guthrie, H. A. 1975. *Introductory Nutrition*. 3rd ed. C. V. Mosby, St. Louis.

Harrison, G. A., J. S. Weiner, J. M. Tanner, N. A. Barnicot, and V. Reynolds. 1977. *Human Biology*. 2nd ed. Oxford University Press.

Hartmann, E. 1967. *The Biology of Dreaming*. Charles C. Thomas Publishers, Springfield, Illinois.

Jacobson, E. 1962. *You Must Relax*. 4th ed. McGraw-Hill Book Co., New York.

Jaffe, D. T. 1980. *Healing from Within*. Alfred A. Knopf, New York.

Katch, F. I. and W. D. McArdle. 1977. *Nutrition, Weight Control, and Exercise*. Houghton Mifflin Co., Boston.

Kleitman, N. 1963. *Sleep and Wakefulness*. University of Chicago Press, Chicago.

Kohn, R. R. 1971. *Principles of Mammalian Aging*. Prentice-Hall, Inc., Englewood Cliff, New Jersey.

Krause, M. V. and L. K. Mahan. 1979. *Food, Nutrition and Diet Therapy*. 6th ed. W. B. Saunders Co., Philadelphia.

Kushi, M. 1977. *The Book of Macrobiotics*. Japan Publications, Inc., Tokyo.

Kushi, M. et al. 1982. *Cancer and Heart Disease: The Macrobiotic Approach to Degenerative Disorders, E. Esko, editor*. Japan Publications, Inc., Tokyo.

Lappé, F. M. 1975. *Diet for a Small Planet*. Ballantine Books, New York.

LeShan, L. 1976. *How to Meditate*. Bantam Books, New York.

Levi, L. (editor). 1967. *Stress: Sources, Management, and Prevention*. Liveright Publishing Corp., New York.

Levy, J. V. and P. Bach-y-Rita. 1976. *Vitamins: Their Use and Abuse*. Liveright Publishing Corp., New York.

Lewin, Sherry. 1976. *Vitamin C, Its Molecular Biology and Medical Potential*. Academic Press, New York.

Lewis, D. H. and R. F. Del Maestro (editors). 1980. "*Free radicals in Medicine and Biology.*" *Acta Physiologica Scandinavica*, Supplement 492.

Luce, G. G. and J. Segal. 1967. *Sleep*. Lancer Books, Inc., New York.

Maharishi Mahesh Yogi. 1969. *On the Bhagavad-Gita: A New Translation and Commentary, Chapters 1–6*. Penguin Books, Inc., Baltimore, Maryland.

March, D. C. 1976. *Handbook: Interactions of Selected Drugs with Nutritional Status in Man*. American Dietetic Association, Chicago.

Mayer, J. 1968. *Overweight: Causes, Cost and Control*. Prentice-Hall, Inc., Englewood Cliffs, New Jersey.

Mayer, J. 1972. *Human Nutrition: Its Physiological, Medical and Social Aspects*. Charles C. Thomas Publishers, Springfield, Illinois.

Mayer, J. 1975. *A Diet for Living*. D. McKay Co., New York.

McLaren, D. S. 1972. *Nutrition and Its Disorders*. Williams and Wilkins Co, Baltimore, Maryland.

Minuchin, S., L. Baker and B. Rosman. 1978. *Psychosomatic Families*. Harvard University Press, Cambridge, Massachusetts.

Mishra, Rammurti S. 1963. *The Textbook of Yoga Psychology*. The Julian Press, Inc. Publishers, New York.

Mitchell, H. S. et al. 1968. *Cooper's Nutrition in Health and Disease*. 15th ed. J. B. Lippincott Co., Philadelphia.

Nakamura, T. 1981. *Oriental Breathing Therapy*. Japan Publications, Inc., Tokyo.

Orme-Johnson, D. W., L. H. Domash and J. T. Farrow (editors). 1974. *Scientific Research on Transcendental Meditation: Collected Papers*. MIU Press, Los Angeles.

Packard, V. S. Jr. 1976. *Processed Foods and the Consumer: Additives, Labeling, Standards and Nutrition*. University of Minnesota Press, Minneapolis.

Pauling Linus. 1976. *Vitamin C, the Common Cold, and the Flu*. W. H. Freeman and Co., San Francisco.

Pike, R. L. and M. L. Brown. 1975. *Nutrition: An Integrated Approach*. 2nd ed. John Wiley & Sons, New York.

Rockstein, M. (editor). 1974. *Theoretical Aspects of Aging*. Academic Press, New York.

Rosa, K. R. 1976. *You and Autogenic Training*. Saturday Review Press/E. P. Dutton, New York.

Ross, D. M. and S. A. Ross. 1976. *Hyperactivity: Research, Theory, and Action*. John Wiley & Sons, New York.

Samuels, M. and N. Samuels. 1976. *Seeing with the Mind's Eye*. Random House/Bookworks, New York.

Selye, H. 1956. *The Stress of Life*. McGraw-Hill Book Co., New York.

Selye. H. 1974. *Stress without Distress*. Signet, New York.

Serban, G. (editor). 1975. *Nutrition and Mental Functions*. Plenum Press, New York.

Serino, G. S. 1966. *Your Ulcer: Prevention, Control, Cure*. J. B. Lippincott Co., Philadelphia.

Simic, M. G. and M. Karel. 1980. *Autoxidation in Food and Biological Systems*. Plenum Press, New York.

Sivananda, Swami. 1929. *Practice of Yoga*. Ganesh and Co., Madras, India.

Sivananda, Swami. 1975. *Concentration and Meditation*. The Divine Life Society, Himalayas, India.

Small, A. E. 1855. *Manual of Homoeopathic Practice for the Use of Families and Private Individuals*. 3rd ed. Rademacher and Sheek, Philadelphia.

Smith, P. 1980. *Total Breathing*. McGraw-Hill Book Co., New York.

Strehler, B. L. 1971. *Aging at the Cellular Level. In: Clinical Geriatrics. I. Rossman, editor*. J. B. Lippincott Co., Philadelphia.

Strehler, B. L. 1977. *Time, Cells, and Aging*. 2nd ed. Academic Press, New York.

Stunkard, A. J. 1976. *The Pain of Obesity*. Bull Publishing Co., Palo Alto, California.

Sussman, Vic S. 1978. *The Vegetarian Alternative*. Rodale Press, Inc., Emmaus, Penn.

Turner, D. 1970. *Handbook of Diet Therapy*. 5th ed. University of Chicago Press, Chicago.

Vishnudevananda, Swami. 1960. *The Complete Illustrated Book of Yoga*. Bell Publishing Co., Inc., New York.

Vivekananda, Swami. 1955. *Raja Yoga*. The Ramakrishna-Vivekananda Center, New York.

Walford, R. L. 1969. *The Immunologic Theory of Aging*. Williams & Wilkins Co., Baltimore, Maryland.

Watanabe, T. and A. Kishi. 1982. *The Book of Soybeans: Nature's Miracle Protein*. Japan Publications, Inc., Tokyo.

Wertheimer, M. 1959. *Productive Thinking*. Harper & Row, Publishers, New York.

Wiener, J. 1970. *Victory through Vegetables*. Holt, Rinehart and Winston, New York.

Winick, M. (editor). 1975. *Childhood Obesity*. John Wiley & Sons, New York.

Wolff, H. G. 1968. *Stress and Disease*. 2nd ed. Charles C. Thomas Publishers, Springfield, Illinois.

Wurtman, Judith J. 1979. *Eating Your Way Through Life*. Raven Press, New York.

Zurbel, R. and V. Zurbel. 1978. *The Vegetarian Family*. Prentice-Hall, Inc., Englewood Cliffs, New Jersey.

Index

Recipe Index

Yoga Postures Index